Their Cancer –

Your Journey

A Traveller's Guide for Carers,

Family and Friends

Anne Orchard

British Library Cataloguing in Publication Data
A Catalogue record for this book is available from The British Library.

ISBN Number: 978-0-9559797-0-5

First edition published by:
Rainbow Heart Publishing
PO Box 7077
Charmouth
BRIDPORT
DT6 9DA
United Kingdom

Telephone: 0844 35 77 959
Website: www.rainbowheartpublishing.co.uk

Note/Disclaimer: The material contained in this book is set out in good faith for general guidance and no liability can be accepted for loss or expense incurred in relying on the information given. In particular this book is not intended to replace competent medical advice. The author is not a medical practitioner, and such advice should be sought if desired before embarking on any health-related program.

To Barbara Lomax and May Orchard:

Two Mums whose very different experiences of cancer

created my journey.

Contents

Acknowledgements and Permissions

The inspiration for this book came from many sources. Firstly my two Mums, who I did my best to support through their illnesses. Next came Blythe House Hospice, and particularly all the ladies of the networking group. Also the Mouth and Foot Painting Artists' Association, who sent me their book by coincidence.

I was fortunate that my wonderful coach Marleen Payne then stayed with me through the wandering until I finally realised the book I really wanted to write.

For the creation of the book I am indebted to Susan Page and Jean-Marie Stine, whose books I consulted at length. I am also grateful to Sue Lascelles who gave much advice at an early stage. I would like to thank Maureen Surgey for her input into the part of the book dealing with bereavement. My editor Jill Greenway has been invaluable, and I could not have published the book without my mentor Linda Parkinson-Hardman showing me the way. Special mention must also go to Steve Graham for putting me in touch with Linda, and for believing in me and my project – you challenged me to act bigger.

For my personal development I would like to thank Robert Allen and Mark Victor Hansen, T. Harv Eker and Peak Potentials, the trainers of CTI UK and my fellow students in Journey 13. It's been a lot of fun!

I would also like to express my gratitude to my father, Jeff Lomax who patiently went through my writing in spite of the emotional content. Last but by no means least I appreciate the support of my husband Pete (which extends beyond encouragement to the creation and maintenance of our websites), and my boys for not complaining too much when their Mum was writing.

I am grateful to CPP for permission to quote passages from the book Co-Active Coaching, and to Julie Blue for permission to reprint the lyrics of her song "Wing And A Prayer" in Chapter 9.

Foreword

This will prove an invaluable book with sensible advice for people who are in the midst of their worst nightmare.

Each chapter deals with a different aspect relating to a diagnosis of cancer. Great advice with special relevance for me, is in Chapter 11- Turn it into Something Good.

John's death was a tragedy. He was a fit, healthy, happy family man, with a great sense of humour; who was highly amused when I joked about an alternative WI calendar, featuring the crafts of WI, but in the nude. Initially, I imagined producing the calendar during his recovery. He was only ill for 5 months and after his death I was determined that we would do the calendar in his memory and raise funds for Leukaemia Research Fund, never envisaging the huge response.

John's wife, Angela says she doesn't know how she would have survived without the calendar. It filled a void and gave her a purpose. We know John has been chuckling, sitting at his desk in Heaven, helping us along.

This book will help and inspire people struggling with cancer to have a positive focus.

Tricia Stewart, Calendar Girl.

Tricia was inspired by the illness of her friend's husband, John Baker, and turned his death into a lasting memorial with her fundraising.

When Cancer Came To Call

There was no sign or warning
No writing on the wall
A day like any other …
When cancer came to call

It grew inside your body
A tumour, starting small
In time the doctor told you
That cancer came to call

I fight against the knowing
"It can't be true," I bawl
But I can't mend you, though I try
For cancer came to call

The things I thought were certain
Seen in my 'crystal ball'
Now lay, hopes dashed and broken
Since cancer came to call

I let go of my feelings
Let all my barriers fall
I must make my own journey
As cancer came to call

I work with my emotions,
The message from them all
Allows me my own healing,
Glad cancer came to call

A sense of peace comes on me
I am as one with all
My love for you is deeper
Now cancer came to call

And as my life moves forwards
I find I'm standing tall
My days are filled with meaning
Since cancer came to call

© 2008, Anne Orchard

1

WHAT WILL YOU GET
FROM THIS BOOK?

Why do you need to read this book? There's nothing wrong with you – it's someone else who has been diagnosed with cancer, after all!

Well, I guess that just sums up the problem. Someone else is ill, but it affects you too. Your life is changing, possibly in a physical way, almost certainly in an emotional one.

You may tell yourself that how you feel isn't important – but that doesn't help anyone. You are a vital and precious person, and you deserve to take some time to travel through this book. You don't *need* to read this book, but you may choose to use it as your guide.

Let's take some time to look at some of the problems you may meet on your journey with another's illness, and some of the ways that this book can help.

Acknowledgement of a Stressful Time

When someone else has cancer, how you feel can seem to pale into insignificance. Everything becomes about the person who is ill. If you were a machine, then you would feel totally neutral about the situation. None of us is built that way, though. We feel deeply, especially when something bad happens to those we care about. I'm glad humans are this way. I wouldn't like to live in a world where nobody had regard for anyone else and how they were feeling.

Being made of flesh and blood (plus an active mind and a vivid imagination) brings its challenges, though. That imagination is where our feelings of stress come from. From fear and worry about the future. When you are dealing with what is happening in the present moment, there is no room for stress. You simply get on and cope with whatever is put before you.

Perhaps this is the first time someone close to you has had cancer, as it was for me when my mother was ill. In this case you may know little of what to expect, and this will almost certainly produce fears of the unknown.

On the other hand, you might have been in a similar situation before, in which case all the emotions you felt then will probably be re-triggered. The challenges you faced in the past become hurdles you expect to have to get over again, even though all cancers and all people are different and so the hurdles will be different too.

Either way, most of the stress you feel is to do with what you fear will happen tomorrow or after many tomorrows. This doesn't make the stress any less real for you right now. There are ways to deal with that stress. The first is simply to notice how much of it is to do with what's happening right now, and how much of it relates to what may or may not happen in the future. Mark Twain famously said "I've had thousands of problems in my life – most of which never actually happened."

You can start your thinking about your loved one's cancer by letting go of as many of those future issues as you can. This will give you some emotional respite, which will allow you then to cope better with the road ahead.

Finding Ways to Protect Your Health

Health is a precious thing. We rarely even realise how precious it is until it is threatened. All the riches in the world are worth little, however, if we don't have the health to enjoy them. You may think I am stating the obvious: your loved one's health is under threat so you are well aware of this issue. Stop for a moment. I'm asking you to consider your own health. Is that difficult? It may feel wrong to be thinking of your own health when your loved one is in such peril right now, but you are under stress.

This will probably be one of the most challenging experiences you ever go through in your life. If you don't look after yourself now, it could threaten your own health in the future. The science of psychoneuroimmunology (PNI for short) is now showing that our state of mind has even more effect on our physical health than has ever been recognised before.

There is a centre in the UK where those with cancer go for

holistic treatment and a more empowered approach to tackling their cancer called Penny Brohn Cancer Care (PBCC). PBCC asked people with cancer what traumatic event in their past they felt had the most effect on their health. Many of them said it had been caring for someone who was ill - either with cancer or another illness. This isn't to say that carers necessarily go on to get cancer. It's just saying that many of those who do get cancer have been affected by someone else's illness in the past.

The good news is that this is now being recognised. PBCC themselves changed their policy as a result. Originally supporters were welcomed to the centre only in that role – to support the person with cancer. Now, though, they are encouraged to go in their own right. They can benefit from the same counselling and treatments as the person with cancer.

You may not choose, or be able, to go on a course at PBCC, but you *can* look after your own health. This will be both a physical and an emotional process. Begin by recognising that your health is also important. Just because you don't have cancer, this doesn't mean you are invulnerable. You can appreciate how precious your health is, and take steps to protect or improve it. In doing this you won't be taking anything away from your loved one.

It isn't wrong to look after yourself when they are struggling; if nothing else you are showing a good example to everyone around you. Also, it could be supportive if you were to join the person who has cancer in some changes to their health regime – even though that's not the main reason for doing so.

Time to step back into your own shoes now. You can see that it is much better for you to be in charge of your own journey, and it is also better for the person who has cancer.

You may be stepping along a path that meanders close to theirs – but your path will have different fears, feelings and challenges. Whilst they may fear dying, for instance, that will relate to what they feel they will miss out on, how painful it may be, or how others will cope with their death. For you, the fear is of losing them – which is very different.

You cannot take the journey for the person who has cancer – and they can't make your journey for you. The two of you may choose to travel together, though, and gain mutual support from doing so. Try not to resist the journey you have to make. You may not have chosen it, but it is yours all the same.

There are probably many other people who care about the person who has cancer, too. Recognise that they all have their own journeys as well. It isn't your job to make those either.

There are many benefits to taking this journey, as you will learn in the rest of the book. Don't deny others their opportunity to gain those benefits as well.

Finding Help for You Too

For many there is a perception that it is only the cancer 'patient' who needs treatment and extra support. Gradually, though, the needs of supporters are being recognised, as I described about PBCC above. Some are beginning to ask the question "Who supports the supporters?" More help is being made available through places like

PBCC, hospices and organisations such as Macmillan Cancer Support in the UK and Cancer*Care* in the USA.

Help is available for you, but in order to get it you will need to ask. Begin by helping yourself as best you can by reading, absorbing and acting on the information in this book. Once you have done this, you will recognise more clearly what help you could use. Half the battle is accepting not only that can you benefit from extra help, but also that you deserve it. Once you can accept that it doesn't make you a bad or weak person to ask for help, you will be able to do so from a good position.

Make a start now by writing down what your biggest issue or challenge is at the moment. This could be anything from not having anyone to talk things over with, to worries about childcare while you go to hospital appointments with your loved one.

Once you know what the issue is you can then move on to what would help you. Write this down; then find someone to ask for this specific help. Most of us find it much easier to respond to a request for exactly what someone needs than to offer general help. For one thing, people often worry whether their offers of help will cause offence.

Don't expect anyone to guess what you need – tell them!

Look For the Positive Side

I'm sure your first reaction is that there couldn't possibly be a positive side to a cancer diagnosis. People who have had cancer tell a different story. With the best support, and particularly if they take their own emotional journey, they often look back and appreciate what they have gained from having cancer. I know no one would volunteer to be in their shoes – or yours. There are certainly much easier ways to gain the same benefits. However, I'm not prepared to agree that a diagnosis of cancer is altogether a bad thing.

As you go through this book, you will find a new way to look at a journey with cancer – both yours and your loved one's. You will learn ways to face up to the worst and then concentrate on what is good in life. You will get to deepen your communication with those you love, and live life more in the present.

It's fine if you're not able to make the leap straight away to accepting the cancer as neutral, rather than an enemy. For the moment, just consider that as a possibility.

Maybe an example would help. I was told of a lady, Amy, who had a stomach tumour that could not be removed by surgery. Rather than fighting the cancer, she worked on imagining it surrounded by a fluffy feather bed – she cosseted it instead! With this 'treatment' the cancer stopped growing, and Amy lived well past the original estimate of the time she had left. She might not have achieved this if she was judging the cancer as a 'bad thing'; that would have meant treating it as an enemy, rather than a part of her body which needed healing.

Strengthen Your Ability to Support

Having your own worries and fears saps your strength. It makes you focus more on yourself, and lessens your ability to reach out to others. How can you keep on giving, if you have no reserves to give from? Eventually you will find yourself running on empty. If you are wrapped up in your own issues, this can make you reactive – you will respond to others from a place of fear rather than compassion and understanding. On the other hand, if you deal with your issues, if you ask for and get the help you need, then you will have much more to give.

There may be many people to whom you can offer support – if you have a surplus of strength. Increasing your capacity to support others is only one reason to work on your own issues, but it may give you the incentive to do so.

Let's face it; there are going to be some tough times ahead, and challenging issues. You may at times feel reluctant to face up to the problems. If being there for others is one motivation you use, then all well and good. Just remember that the main reason for sorting yourself out is for your benefit – being able to support others is just one of the things that you might gain.

Create a Better Outcome – Whatever the Outcome

I wish I could tell you now what the outcome will be of your loved one's cancer – but nobody can do that. You can't yet see the end of the journey. In many cases this could be a blessing, as it allows you to deal with reality as you find it today. The actions you take (or don't) today may affect the eventual outcome of your loved one's journey with cancer. At this time, no one can say. Even if you can't control the end result of their disease, you can control your own experience of it.

By buying this book, you have taken an enormous first step. By reading and using it you will be more in control than most people in a similar situation. By participating fully in the journey you can learn from the experience and grow with those around you. When you reach your destination you will be in better shape. You will have learned and practised new skills and coping strategies. You will then be able to build on the relationship you have with the person who has cancer – or else be better equipped to build a life without that person.

Hope For the Future

One of the things that will keep you going in the days and months ahead is hope. Never lose sight of hope. Robert Louis Stevenson said, "It is better to travel hopefully than to arrive." This may not be true for you if your destination is one of joy, but you don't know right now, so travelling hopefully is sound advice.

You will find as you read that I ask you to face up to unpleasant possibilities – this is really so that you can understand what is going on. Face your fears, rather than hiding them and worrying in secret. Even while you do that, you can still keep hope with you.

There may be times when you feel that life will never get better – particularly if you are faced with a poor outlook for your loved one's cancer. In this case, you can still find realistic things to hope for. If your loved one is unlikely to get better, you can hope they find peace. You can hope for relief from pain, and above all you can hope for everyone to find meaning in the experience. There is always something to hope for, and living in hope is the life to choose.

Sharing the Lessons

If you have picked up this book, it is likely that your experience of someone else's cancer is happening right now. If not, there could still be a benefit in reading it and making sense of a cancer that happened in your past.

For me, that experience began many years ago. My mother was diagnosed with secondary brain tumours at the very beginning of 1991. At Christmas we had been aware that there was something wrong, especially that Mum was having a lot of headaches, but it took a little time to get the actual diagnosis. Mum died later that same year, and the rest of the family pulled through as best we could. We didn't think deeply about what we had been through (or at least I didn't at the time), and we all coped separately.

As the years went by, however - as I learned and grew as a person - more of the experience began to make sense to me. I found a feeling of peace about what had happened. I have reached a place where I truly feel it is fine that my mother died of cancer. Maybe this seems very unlikely to you now, but it is a peaceful way to feel. It doesn't take anything away from how hard the experience was at the time, but it does mean that there was some point to it all.

Many years later my mother-in-law also had cancer – this time diagnosed after a routine mammogram. I am sure that the support I was able to offer her was much stronger because of the work I had already done relating to my mother's illness. I am glad to be able to tell you that my mother-in-law came through her cancer and is still well as I write this book.

You can see that I have been through two very different experiences with loved ones having cancer, and this gives me some perspective – but it's only my perspective.

In this book I will share much of what I learned, and tell

some stories about my experiences and those of others. You will read those stories through the filters of what you are going through. They may mean something different for you than they did for me. That is just fine.

I invite you to take this journey for yourself. If what I say makes sense to you, then take it on board. If it doesn't seem right to you at first, just try the ideas on for size. See if life looks better or worse with a new point of view. Keep whatever works for you, and just let go of the rest. What you gain from this book is entirely up to you. I am happy just to let my lessons go out into the world to see if they can help others. I hope you will do the same with your own lessons.

This may not be an easy journey, but it is your journey, and your own attitude will determine how that journey goes.

A Final Word on How to Use This Book

Most books are designed to be read straight through from start to finish – and of course you can read this book the same way if you like. You might want to take it more slowly, though. Your journey may be over quickly, or it may stretch out over time. If yours is an extended journey, you may find it best to concentrate on the parts of the book that are relevant to you now.

This is definitely not a book to read and then forget about. It is packed with suggestions of ways you can improve your situation, and it would be challenging to put them all into action at one time. Here is how I suggest you will get the most out of your reading:

- Send an email to sendwb@familiesfacingcancer.org. This will then give you a link to download a free workbook with space to answer some questions and get more out of this book as you go through it. If you don't have computer access, ask someone to get this for you.

- Read the chapters that are relevant now, or cover stages of your journey that are in the past. At the end of each chapter you will find a single action step, so take just this one step. (You can start with the one at the end of this chapter!)

- Once you have done that, go back and read the parts that are relevant at the current stage of your journey again. See what additional actions you might want to add in. In this way you will get more out of the book each time you read it.

- As you continue on your journey, new chapters will become relevant, so visit them when they will help you most.

- Please also visit our website. I set up the organisation Families Facing Cancer to back up the information in this book, and it seems to be developing a life of its own. At **www.familiesfacingcancer.org**, you can join a community of fellow travellers and make sure you're not on your own – even though your journey is individual to you, there's nothing wrong with having a little support on the road.

ACTION STEP

Think about what your intention is in reading this book. What do you want to achieve by reading it? How do you hope to feel at the end? You already know what my intention was in writing it, but that doesn't matter.

You don't have to ponder it for a long time. Just write down the first thing that comes into your head. Simply by setting your intention, you will have given your subconscious mind the task of looking for what you need in these pages. I trust you will find it.

2

THE UNEXPECTED BEGINNING OF THE JOURNEY

You may have heard that every journey begins with a single step. In fact a journey usually begins before a step has been taken. It begins when the *decision* is made to take that first step. For the journey at the heart of this book, that choice was made for you. The decision has been made by the diagnosis.

Shock of Diagnosis

Somehow a diagnosis of cancer always manages to be a shock. Even if it was your worst fear, the chances are you will still feel shocked to hear the word. You may hear the diagnosis after a long period of uncertainty. Maybe your loved one has been ill for some time, and you have not been able to find out what was wrong before. Perhaps the cancer was found during a routine screening, and was the last thing anyone expected. You may have been with your friend or relative when they were told, or have received a telephone call out of the blue. However you heard, and however expected (or not) the diagnosis was, you are likely to have had a physical reaction.

Human minds are not very good at distinguishing between types of peril. Your body will respond in much the same way to a cancer diagnosis as it would to a tiger on the horizon. Both are scary prospects! This is known as the 'fight or flight' response. Your body makes adrenaline in response to your thoughts. The result of this is to increase blood flow to your limbs in order to make you ready for action. Because blood is diverted away from your brain, it reduces your ability to think clearly. So don't be surprised if later you can't remember any detail of what you have been told. Many people report that they can't recall a single word that was said to them after the word 'cancer'.

When the adrenaline reaction dies down, you may then feel tired or depressed. This is understandable from an emotional point of view. However, it is made worse by the physical reaction caused by the adrenaline. You feel drained and don't know how you are going to cope. Try to take heart that you will find a way. Be kind and understanding to yourself.

The Journey is Forced Upon You

Many journeys are chosen. There is the excitement of planning, or possibly a decision to make a change. Not this time. This situation is more like a natural disaster. A volcano has erupted in your life – and you are fleeing from its effects. You have no time to stop and collect your belongings, and certainly no choice in the matter. You are simply moving. Everything familiar has been left behind.

You are probably filled with unanswered questions. Where and when will the journey end? Nobody can tell for sure. Even if you have been told the likely outcome of the disease, there will be a range of possibilities, or timescales. Your final destination is clouded in mystery.

You may even call into question your own health. Most people tend to take this for granted in their everyday lives. You probably take some exercise or make good choices about what you eat. When you've done that, however, the chances are that you will rely on your body being there for you, allowing you to do what needs to be done. This proof, which shows up the uncertainty that health will continue, can bring in doubts. You wonder how long your own health will last.

This is a perfectly normal reaction – and it doesn't make you selfish or uncaring. You will find in the days, weeks and months ahead you will have many thoughts and feelings you don't like. Be easy on yourself. You were never prepared for this. There wasn't a course at school entitled 'Coping When Someone Else Gets Ill'! You are starting from scratch, like everyone else who took a similar journey. You will learn as you go along. Those thoughts you believe are ungracious or that you 'shouldn't' have are not something to be ashamed of. They are perfectly natural reactions. These thoughts may even contain messages you need to take into account. You are not responsible for your thoughts – only for how you react to them.

No One Plans to Get Cancer!

Of course, it is obvious that no one plans to get cancer, but that is also something you can forget.

Consider for a moment the person who has been handed this diagnosis. It doesn't matter what life choices they have made up to this point. Whether they ate unhealthy food, didn't take care of their bodies or even smoked – it is very unlikely that they made these life choices with the intention of getting cancer!

You may even have heard or read about the 'Cancer Personality', and think that it was to be expected that your loved one would find themselves in this position. There may even be a trace of truth in this, but if so they will still not have made a conscious choice.

What does this mean for you? It means that if you find those thoughts arising – for instance, "Well, what did they expect, smoking for all those years?" – it is important to set them aside.

You won't be the only person to think those things. You may even find other people say them to you, including perhaps the person who has cancer. But those choices are, and can only stay, in the past. They are irrelevant. The only thing that matters is what choices you make now. Don't play the blame game, either with your own thoughts or with anyone else who raises the subject.

Don't Blame the Messenger

You can also be tempted to apply the blame game to outside factors. Pollution, government, mobile phone masts, the medical profession perhaps for not making the diagnosis sooner), God, or even the cancer itself may become the objects of your fury.

It's always appealing to look for someone or something to take responsibility for the situation. The truth is, though, that even if you know whose fault it is, anger doesn't serve you.

A more helpful approach is to treat the cancer as a messenger. At the simplest level, it brings a message that some part of your loved one is hurting and needs to be healed. There may be an influence in their life or in society that has contributed, and so the message may be that something needs to change.

On a deeper level, there may be a message that something is wrong emotionally that your loved one can fix (though this still doesn't mean they are to blame for their cancer). For instance Penny Brohn Cancer Care (the Centre I mentioned in Chapter 1) works on a holistic principle. That means the best help for cancer involves treating any ailing emotions of the person, as well as their body. They need to heal in more than one way.

Losing the Victim Label

How do you see your loved one, now that they have cancer? They have become part of the statistics – 'one in three people get cancer at some point in their lives'; '280,000 cancer diagnoses in the UK every year'. Does this in some way weaken them in your eyes?

We live today in a society where the people in trouble are always treated as victims. You see it in the headlines. The word 'Victim' sells newspapers. It is also part of the blame game we discussed already, as there can only be a *victim* if someone or something is to blame. So the chances are that society has made you inclined to feel sorry for this person.

So deep-rooted is this attitude that I am struggling to find a word to describe this person who has the cancer in their body in a way that does not almost pity them. Traditionally we say 'the cancer patient' (which implies they are the passive receiver of treatment), 'the cancer sufferer' (poor them), or worst of all, 'the cancer victim'. Can you see how negative these are? If this is the way you think of your loved one, it will colour every contact you have with them.

I went to great efforts to find a more positive description. I asked my local hospice what term they use. They understood the problem perfectly. The term they use is their 'guests', as that seems so much more neutral. My husband made up the term 'canceree', but it seemed too artificial. My sister suggested 'the cancer host', and that seems the best so far. If you ignore thoughts of parasites, then you can treat the cancer as a rather unwelcome guest to which your loved one is playing host - at least for the time being.

You may even think of a better term, but see what works for you. The person you care about is still there. They have been given a challenge, and will probably appreciate your support. But they are still a whole person. You will do them an immense favour by treating them as this.

Don't tread on eggshells. Believe in their ability to cope with what life throws at them. Weep with them, but not for them. Laugh with them, too. They will discover reserves they never knew they had, and so will you.

Grieving For the 'Expected' Life

There are many events life throws at us which involve big changes. When you look at a list of the most stressful events in life they include such things as bereavement, divorce and moving house. The stress involved in moving house is mostly due to uncertainty – will problems arise before the sale is finished? This uncertainty is also a feature of the situation you find yourself in, and you will find ways to help you to deal with this later in the book.

In fact all these events have an element of loss in common. When you are bereaved you are grieving for a person (or the loss of your life relationship with that person). When a relationship ends through divorce or split, you are grieving for the loss of what that meant in your life. When someone is diagnosed with cancer, you are grieving for the loss of the life you expected to have in relation to them. That carefree life of opportunity and health is on hold for the time being. It is natural to feel sad or angry about that.

It may be that when the cancer is diagnosed, you are told that there is a poor outlook. In this case you may begin the grieving process for the death of that person ahead of time. This is covered in much more depth in Chapter 9, Arriving Part 2: Adjusting To Loss.

When my mother was diagnosed with secondary brain tumours, there was little treatment possible. In the initial adjustment I was grieving for the loss of things in our relationship at that moment. For instance, she was unable to carry on writing a letter every fortnight to update us on what was going on in our siblings' lives. I missed those letters.

I was also grieving for the fact that she might not be around in the future. I had been expecting to have many discussions (and disagreements) with her about bringing up my children. Children were still in my future, but my mother might not be – I didn't know for sure.

Expected Life is an Illusion

No one can tell you what tomorrow holds. I would give good odds, though, that you have been telling yourself what you *thought* the future would bring. I once had a miscarriage at an early stage; I had known I was pregnant for less than two weeks. Not very long at all. It was, however, plenty long enough to have built a fantasy life around that child – ranging all the way from breastfeeding to graduation from college! So when I lost the baby, much of my sadness was because of this fantasy.

I now have two boys, and I can tell you that life is nothing like the rose-tinted illusion I painted all that time ago. I had made the experience much harder for myself by my flights of fancy.

Now this is an extreme example, but we all do much the same in our daily lives. You probably know what pastimes you are looking forward to in retirement – delayed for years, perhaps, while you do 'what must be done' to earn a living. If you are already retired, perhaps your future illusions are of many more years stretching ahead with little change.

Now you have found yourself in a situation that shows these illusions up for what they are – castles in the air! You now don't know what the future holds, which of course was really the situation all along. In the words of the old song "I beg your pardon – I never promised you a rose garden". Nobody promised you that your fantasies would come true. Painful though it will be, now is the time to let go of the attachment you have to the visions you have created.

Some of those visions may still be of use to you, though. You could have a trip you have been delaying, or something you planned to do with your loved one some day in the future. That could give a useful focus – something to look forward to. It is important not to be too attached to the outcome, though. You no longer have the luxury of that illusion of certainty. What is valuable is to enjoy the process. My husband's aunt enjoyed looking forward to a trip to New Zealand to visit her son. Thinking about that holiday gave her so much pleasure that it was worth doing, even though she was never well enough to make the trip.

Death is a Natural Part of Life

You may be wondering why I'm talking about death at this early stage of the book. After all, your loved one has only just been diagnosed. Surely it's far too negative to mention death at this point? It's unlikely (unless you have received a very late diagnosis) that the medical team has raised the prospect of death. However there is a big 'But' to consider. Many advances have been made in the field of cancer treatment; but it is still something that people die from. In fact, as our ability to treat other conditions improves, it becomes ever more common that cancer is what will finally take us out of this world.

This means that whenever the word cancer is mentioned, the thought of the chance of death comes swiftly after. You will probably be trying to suppress it. You have almost certainly heard of the benefits of positive thinking, and want to apply it. The trouble is that the little voice in your head that says "What if they die?" is not easy to silence. The more you push it down, and refuse to listen to it, the stronger it is likely to become. I'm not telling you it's a good idea to dwell on the likelihood of your loved one's death. I'm just saying you need to acknowledge that thought.

The truth is that death is certain for all of us. It's a natural part of life. You can think of it as being like the passing of the seasons. Our birth and death are as woven into the fabric of nature as the growth and falling of leaves on the trees each year. Cancer is by no means an inevitable death sentence, but we all have to go eventually. Who can say how long we are supposed to be here?

If your loved one's cancer does lead to death (either now or in many years' time), there is no point in resisting this. Yes, you will do everything in your power to support them and their health, but if that proves to be to no avail, so be it.

Children have a very practical attitude to death. They feel the grief and sadness as deeply as we do, they just don't let it linger. They understand instinctively that life goes on. Once their grief has been expressed and noticed by others, they are likely to switch rapidly to getting on with the business of their lives, such as playing with their friends. They have a natural approach.

Society's attitude has a great influence on our perception of death. Only a hundred years ago, most families would have experienced death first hand. Children died in infancy, mothers died in childbirth. In my husband's family, his great grandfather was given the same name as another baby who died only a year before. This would be unthinkable now, but I think it shows how naturally death was treated then – because it was more common.

These days we have removed death from the family and into hospitals. The result is that it has become surrounded by an air of mystery. It also seems that death is almost always regarded with horror – instead of as a natural stage which we would all welcome at some point in our lives.

Other societies have different attitudes. In ancient Celtic cultures, for instance, they believed (as do many people today) that the person who dies moves on to something greater. They celebrated death for the person they loved. In their culture a birth was a time for mourning, as they felt that the spirit of the child had lost their freedom by becoming restricted to our physical world.

So do not fear death. Or if you are feeling fear, notice what is at the root of the fear. Are you afraid of being lonely, or of a lack of support? Would you desperately miss spending time with a person who brings joy into your life? Be honest with yourself, face up to your fears, and you will do much to still that little voice. This will then allow you to give more concentration to what you can do now to help.

As Deepak Chopra said in *The Book of Secrets* "Only by facing death can you develop a real passion for being alive."

How Do Others React?

When facing a cancer diagnosis, one issue you (and the person who has cancer) will face is the attitudes of other people. There are many different ways that others will handle the news. Some may have difficulty talking about the cancer at all. They may go to great lengths to avoid the subject. You may even find that they seem to be avoiding you, or the cancer host.

You may feel very hurt at what seems like indifference or lack of compassion. In fact this behaviour probably shows that they have some unresolved issues that make it hard for them to deal with illness. You may have no idea what has happened in their past for them to behave that way. It may not lessen the hurt you feel, but try not to blame them.

Other people may have a 'poor you' attitude. They will be pitying in the extreme for the 'terrible situation' in which you find yourself. This could feel good in one way. You are getting sympathy for your situation, and it's nice to know that someone has noticed how awful it is! At least they don't think the cancer host is the only person who deserves sympathy. So accept their expression of sympathy the first time. Be especially glad if it is accompanied by genuine offers of practical help or emotional support. But if you find you are on the receiving end of endless streams of pity from some people, be wary. Whilst they may truly care for you, if they belittle your ability to cope with the situation this attitude could rub off on you. Both you and the person with the cancer need to be empowered to deal with the challenges ahead, not brought down to the victim mindset. It may be that you have to tell people, "Thanks for the sympathy, but I know we'll get through this." Possibly you could add, "What you can do to help is . . .". If they continue to be negative, you may choose to limit the time you spend with them.

On the other hand, some people will be absolutely amazing. Firm friendships have appeared seemingly from nowhere in the face of adversity. When my first marriage broke down, my colleague, Jenny, took me into her home while I looked for somewhere to live.

She talked to me as I made difficult decisions for the future and was the most staunch supporter I had at the time. She was a truly lovely person and a deep friendship came out of that experience. So be prepared to be surprised and delighted by how some people come through for you.

The truth of the matter is that other people's reactions are just that – theirs! Whilst it is natural to feel happy or sad about how others behave, the fact is that their reaction is not about you. It relates to who they are, the experiences they have gone through and how they handle issues in their own lives. Don't take it personally. Just make the most of those whose attitude helps you.

Looking at Relationships

It's at times of crisis that you find out what your relationships are made of. Are they strong as steel, rigid and brittle as glass, cloying as treacle, or comfortable and yielding as a squashy couch?

At this time your relationship with the cancer host is likely to be at least examined, if not tested! When someone has cancer, they may not be investing into their emotional bank account with you. There will be other things on their mind. How is that bank account? Is it already overdrawn? If so, you may struggle to offer them support, and feel resentful if they call on you for help. If, on the other hand, you have a strong relationship that you have both been investing in, you will find it easier to deal with the demands ahead.

Whatever has gone before, your relationship will change. I can't predict how it will change, but it will. It could deepen immensely with this experience, or fall apart at the seams. There is much that you can do to affect how your relationship ends up. The most helpful tool you can use will be communication – true, honest, open communication. This is not something that always comes naturally, so you will find it covered in much more depth later, in Chapter 3. If you deal with any issues or disagreements that have kept you apart in the past, you have the opportunity now to build a better relationship for the future.

When my mother was ill, I found it became possible to talk to her about issues I thought would stay secret forever. The reasons I had for keeping those secrets suddenly seemed so trivial in the face of Mum's illness. Even though she later died, it was a great comfort to me that we had mended much of what was wrong with our past relationship.

Your relationships with many other people will also change. The different reactions that you experience from others, as I have already mentioned, will be part of this. You will also affect those relationships – and they will affect you.

Are there relationships that have been draining your energy for some time? Look seriously at whether you want to ease back from them. Can you afford to give your energy to people who offer nothing in return? You may have new demands on your energy now – it is your turn to look for support from the people around you who are able to give it.

This isn't an excuse to collapse and expect others in the family who may also be suffering from the current turmoil to carry the can for you. Instead, you can mutually explore your relationships with others who are also affected by the cancer. The effect of this illness won't necessarily break or fix those relationships – in the same way as having a child can bring parents closer or push them apart. What it will do is add *pressure* to that relationship. It is up to you what results from that pressure.

You can look to those who are less affected to offer you support. It has been truly said that "No man is an island". Love and support from others are some of our most basic needs. Babies who have their physical needs met but do not receive loving contact with other humans are not able to grow and function properly. You still have some of that baby's needs. So don't 'soldier on'. Look at the people in your life, and who can help you.

You may develop your relationships with several people. You could have someone to cry with, someone to go out for a light-hearted chat or to the cinema with, and someone practical who will help you solve the problems that arise. They don't have to all be the same person – in fact it would probably be better if they were not. Allow yourself to be a little vulnerable. See who steps up to be with you at this time.

Friends often feel very hurt when a family closes ranks around an ill person. They cannot understand why they should be shut out, though often this is the wish of the person who is ill. Allowing them to offer their support to you will keep them feeling involved. It will give them the deep satisfaction of being able to do *something*. If you are that friend, offer to help the family even if you can't directly help the cancer host.

Time to Take Stock

Just as others want to do something, anything, to help, your first reaction may be to jump into action. In fact the adrenaline will probably give you that urge. However, your first job is really to adjust to the new situation. Taking action may make you feel better, more in control, but it can also be a cover-up. It can be an excuse for not facing up to the full reality of the situation. That is a dangerous road to go down.

If you suppress your feelings about the diagnosis, that will use up a lot of energy – energy that could be used in much better ways.

Try not to make snap decisions. Everyone needs time to let the reality sink in. Your loved one may be under pressure to make decisions about treatment if the medical team feel that time is of the essence. In this case treatment will probably have started before you are reading these words. But try to step out of the whirlwind for a little while.

You will find lots of ways for processing emotions later in this book (Chapter 6), but for now just jot down some notes:

- How are you feeling?
- What do you know about the situation?
- What do you want to know?
- What are your biggest worries or fears?

This process will allow the reality to sink in a little. It takes time to adjust to a change as big as this, but you can adjust – probably better than you could possibly imagine now.

I often hear people say such things as "I just don't know how he/she coped with that situation." In fact when you have no choice, you can cope with the most extreme realities.

Treat yourself gently now. All emotions are acceptable; just try to make sure your reactions don't adversely affect others. Begin taking steps to de-stress other areas of your life. Become aware if there are any other areas of your life where you have major issues. These will affect your ability to cope with your loved one's cancer, so make sure you're aware of them now.

Reaching Out to Others

How do you usually deal with problems in your life? Do you talk them over with others? Muddle your way through on your own? If your natural style is to get support from other people, you may already have a strong network of friends. But perhaps you have recently moved to a new area and don't know many people. Maybe you are too busy for a full social life and only have acquaintances at work. In this case, it is time to start building your support network now.

You may feel very sensitive, and that you don't want people feeling sorry for you, but don't close yourself off. If you do, you will be missing out on all that others have to offer you – and doing them a disservice.

If you feel uncomfortable approaching and getting to know people, being open to others will be like using a muscle that hasn't been exercised for some time. That's no reason to give up! Keep trying, be open: the first step will be to let people know what is going on in your life.

Expressing How You Feel

One reason you may hold back from talking to people about what's going on in your life is fear. Fear of your own feelings, or of what will happen if you begin to express them! Will you break down and cry? Are you only just holding it together by ignoring the issue for as much of the day as you can?

The truth is you probably need to cry, and may continue to have this need for some time. When you fail to express - or let go of - your emotions they become stuck and this can lead to further problems. The challenge is that this is often not be acceptable in public. Weeping at work, whilst understandable, may not be the best career move. You need a safe space and time to express how you're feeling.

Writing is one way to do this. For some, physical activity will help. If you are feeling furious with life, hammering a squash ball or pushing weights could be therapeutic. A long walk can also give the same benefits. If you have someone with whom you usually talk about your feelings, set aside some time to spend with him or her. Tell them you don't want anything fixing just now, just to let off some steam. More methods for dealing with emotions can be found in Chapter 6: The Inner Journey.

Effect on Your Ability to Function

The beginning of a journey as momentous as that with another's cancer is no small undertaking. People's attitudes to the road ahead are many and varied. There are stoical types who grit their teeth and adopt the 'Blitz' spirit. There are those who fall apart at the mere thought of illness, and cannot imagine how they will cope. There are others who refuse to even think about their loved one's illness, hoping that this means the problem will somehow go away. Then there are the rest of the population, for whom all of these and many more reactions are true – at different times.

When my mother was ill (but we didn't yet know she had cancer) I used to find myself in control one minute and in tears the next. I would be talking to a colleague, and suddenly begin to sob. I thought I was over-reacting to the fact that she might have had a stroke. But this was my Mum. She was ill, and I couldn't control the thoughts that came up in those early days.

As you adjust to your new reality there are some key issues to consider:

- If you are in employment, you need to let someone know the situation. However private a person you are, it is important that your employer is aware of the situation, just in case your work is affected. Most employers will be very understanding in these circumstances.

- If you run your own business, consider whether there are duties that you can delegate. It is important that your business does not suffer, so take steps now to safeguard this. Who knows, you may find a new way of doing things that works even better.

- If you have children who are also affected, let their teachers and other group leaders know what is going on. My friend Emma, who is a Boy Scout group leader, was disciplining a child at her group without realising that his father had died. You do not know how a child's emotions will be affecting their behaviour in the short term; so don't let something like this happen to your child because you find it hard to talk about the situation.

- Domestic chores are another area where you may be able to reduce stress. It isn't a crime to let things slide on the home front for a little while as you adjust to the situation.

Give yourself time to change. You will get used to the new reality, but it is important to be especially kind to yourself in this period of adjustment. Once you accept things as they are, your ability to function normally will gradually improve. You may not return to exactly where you were before the diagnosis, but you will reach a higher level than in the period of shock when you first find out what was wrong.

ACTION STEP

Make a start on expressing your feelings about what is happening. Use any of the following options, whichever one appeals to you most:

1. Draw or paint a picture that expresses something about how you feel.

2. Write a letter, journal entry or poem about the situation. Add colour to your writing to get more in touch with your feelings.

3. Ask someone who is less affected than you to be a listening ear. Make sure you tell them you just want someone to hear how you're feeling, not for them to solve your problem. If you don't have anyone specific to talk to, you could phone a help or advice line of one of the cancer charities. This could also be done online, e.g. at the Macmillan Share forum.

4. Make some time on your own at home and throw a 'hissy fit'. Stamp, scream, throw or punch cushions – whatever lets you release the negative emotions. For this to work, you really have to get into it!

3

LEARNING TO COMMUNICATE

When it comes down to any situation that involves emotions and other people, there are only two skills that make a difference. The first skill is introspection – looking inside yourself at how you feel, and working on what you find. If the truth be told, this is only another form of the second skill – communication.

How well you communicate (both with yourself and with other people) is the single factor that will make the most difference in how well you weather the journey ahead. So even if it seems irrelevant right now, you need to look at this skill and how you can improve it.

First, let's look at why there could be a problem in an area that is so vital. Then we'll move on to how to make things better.

Why Don't We Communicate?

We communicate with other people nearly every day of our lives. We've been doing it since we were small children. Surely we should be pretty good at it by now? Well, we're not!

I assume you've noticed that sometimes people don't get along. The vast majority of problems that arise between relatives, partners, businesses, employees and countries can be boiled down to poor communication.

Why *are* we so bad at communicating? Actually, we have been taught to be! Have you ever encouraged a small child to speak – the "say Dada" phase? Parents and other adults start off by delighting in every word their children utter. Then have you ever been on the receiving end of a torrent of conversation from a four year old? Most of it is barely comprehensible, or is an endless stream of "Why does it/is it/can't I?" type questions.

It is little wonder that, to protect our poor, slow adult brains from the speed at which a child interacts with the world, we go to great lengths to get them to *talk less*. Maybe things are a little better now, but not so long ago it was the expectation that 'children should be seen and not heard'. Did your parents believe that when you were a child? Gradually you stop sharing your feelings, thoughts and insights – because they seem to fall on deaf ears.

The other reason we are poor communicators is that to be good ones we have to really listen to the other person. That isn't as easy as it sounds.

If you are accepted as a volunteer for the Samaritans (who offer telephone support for those thinking of committing suicide), for instance, you have to take a course that includes learning to listen. When couples go to marriage guidance, the first job of the counsellor is to get them each to *hear* what the other person is saying. It may be the first time they have ever done this. When they truly hear how their partner feels, sometimes this on its own is enough to allow them to resolve their differences.

You can see that listening is important. In my life coach training, we studied ways of listening in some detail. I would like to share the insights I gained from that.

Listening Skills

Most of the time we hardly even listen to anyone else at all. Most of our conversations are at a superficial level. When was the last time you feel you talked to someone about the things that really matter in life, rather than about things that have to be done or problems that have occurred?

In order for a meaningful exchange of views to take place, we have to truly hear what the other person is telling us. I will share with you the three levels of listening that I learned from my coaching training, so you can understand how to do this. This description of these levels is taken from the book *Co-Active Coaching* by Laura Whitworth, Karen Kimsey-House, Henry Kimsey-House and Phillip Sandahl.

The interpretations are my own and so any errors are entirely my fault:

➤ Level I – Internal listening

"At Level I, our awareness is on ourselves. We listen to the words of the other person, but our attention is on what it means to us personally. At Level I, the spotlight is on 'me': my thoughts, my judgements, my feelings, my conclusions about myself and others. Whatever is happening to the other person is coming back to us through a diode: a one-way energy trap that lets information in but not out. We're absorbing information by listening but holding it in a trap that recycles it. At Level I, there is only one question: 'What does this mean to me?'"

When you are talking to the cancer host or someone else who is affected, this is the natural level of listening in which to find yourself. The chances are that whatever is said to you, you will have an internal dialogue.

It could go along the lines of "But what about me? I'm under enough stress as it is; I don't need all this." And then perhaps "Oh, what an awful person I must be! Poor them, they have cancer and all I can think about is that I don't have time to look after them as well as everything else."

As I said, it's hardly surprising that we have these thoughts. A cancer diagnosis is a dramatic thing in anyone's life, whether it is you who has cancer, or someone you care about. However, these thoughts take up a lot of your attention. Your mind is then distracted and you will miss much of what is said to you.

It happens to me when I am coaching. When I am having an internal dialogue about what I'm going to say next, my client can tell. They may not realise why, but they will start to ramble, and stop saying anything meaningful. It's very hard to express yourself to a void, which is what you are doing when your words don't arrive anywhere.

What do I do when I find this happening? I admit it! I say "Sorry, I got a bit distracted there, I didn't really hear what you said." I may even share what my dilemma or distraction was. That way I am being authentic, and can get back on track. If I don't do that, my client assumes that there was something 'wrong' about what they were saying. Such is our insecurity!

➢ Level II – Focused listening

"At Level II, there is a sharp focus on the other person. Sometimes you can see it in each person's posture: both leaning forward, looking intently at each other. There is a great deal of attention on the other person and not much awareness of the outside world.

When you are listening at Level II, your awareness is totally on [the other person]. You listen for their words, their expression, their emotions, everything that they bring. You notice what they say, how they say it. You notice what they don't say. You see their smiles or hear the tears in their voices."

From my perspective, Level II listening is very much about connection. To achieve it successfully, it is helpful to stop for a moment and think about moving your focus from yourself to the other person. This isn't a permanent transfer, but it allows you to take in more from the contact you are about to have. You can also do this if you are talking to someone and realise you have slipped into Level I.

The purpose of Level II listening is to allow you to have fuller and more honest communication. For instance you may be with the cancer host. They may be 'putting a brave face on things', but something you pick up in their voice or their face tells you that this isn't the whole truth. Rather than accusing them of anything, you would then ask "I'm getting a funny idea that there's something you're not telling me. You seem afraid of something. What is that?" In Level I you might make a judgement or assumption about that, in Level II you would be open minded and interested in what they have to say. By asking an open question (one that doesn't have a yes/no answer) you can follow up on what they've said, and create a much deeper conversation. It may feel scary if you're not used to talking to this person at such a deep level. It is conversations like these, ones that feel edgy and a bit dangerous, that really make a difference in relationships.

➢ Level III – Global listening

"When you listen at Level III, you listen as though you and the [other person] were at the centre of the universe, receiving information from everywhere at once. It's as though you were surrounded by a force field that contains you, the [other person] and an environment of information. Level III includes everything you can observe with your senses: what you see, hear, smell, and feel – the tactile as well as the emotional sensations. Level III includes the action, the inaction and the interaction."

This is what some might call intuition. If you tap into it, you will gather more information than you can imagine. You can even collect this information without talking to the person involved. Simply think about them, your relationship and the situation you are in. Then sit and write down everything you know about them and your relationship. What is their biggest challenge? How do they view the situation? What are their strengths and how do they make life difficult for themselves. If you do this correctly (and that means putting yourself in their shoes with no judgement), you will learn much about the person. You can then use your hunches, check them out with the person, and again take your communications to a deeper level.

If you're having a hard time understanding this level of 'listening', here is an exercise you can try in order to experience it for yourself. Then you will understand the power much more clearly.

1. Find someone who is willing to try it out with you, then sit facing each other in chairs you can easily move.
2. Look into each other's eyes and feel the connection between you. You may find this uncomfortable and want to giggle, but keep relaxing until you feel a connection.
3. Turn your chairs back to back and sit without touching. Allow yourself to continue feeling the connection.
4. Ask yourself what they are feeling or thinking about.
5. Check out with each other your impressions and see how accurate you were. This is Level III listening.

You may feel as though what you really want is someone to listen to YOU! This might make you reluctant to put energy into listening to others, but there is a point.

Practising these listening skills, although it seems like putting others first, will make it more likely that you will also be heard. By having Level II conversations, and practising your Level III skills, you will break the cycle where people talk, but nothing is really said. When the person you are talking to feels you truly hear them, you may find they are better able to listen to you too. If you still feel that you need someone to listen to you, you can always hire a life coach (more of this later).

Communicating with the Medical Profession

If you are close to the person who has cancer, you may talk directly with the medical team who are caring for them. In addition to doctors, this team may also include others such as therapists and hospice workers. If you wish to communicate with the medical team, but the person with cancer does not want you there, you could feel frustrated. If you find yourself in this situation, all you can do is handle your feelings and make sure you are communicating with the cancer host well. Then you are more likely to get the information you feel you are lacking. Above all respect your loved one's wishes.

There are many different ways that friends and family communicate with the medical team. These depend on both their personality and the emotions they are feeling.

- Some relatives of people who have cancer are aggressive in appointments with doctors. This may be especially the case if they feel there has been an omission or that a diagnosis could have been made sooner. This approach is unlikely to be helpful, however genuine your emotions. The time for dealing with those emotions is not in a short hospital appointment. Your loved one will have little enough time to find out what they need to know. Whilst any major error needs to be dealt with, that should not be allowed to cloud the treatment of the cancer host. It is also not your place to be in charge.

- Some relatives are autocratic, commanding, and even ignore the wishes of the person who has the cancer. This may be a continuation of a pattern in your relationship from before the cancer. If your loved one is to recover, it will help if they feel in charge of themselves and their treatment in some way. It may be tempting to step in – you may feel you know better, or be used to speaking on their behalf – but it is very unlikely to help. It is also tempting for the medical staff to speak to you if you seem to be in charge. But there is nothing more demoralising for a person receiving treatment than to have that treatment discussed with another as if they weren't even there.

- Some people are submissive, treating the medical teams as the ones who are in control and assuming their word is law. There is a fine line to tread here. It may be that the person with cancer needs to trust their medical team completely in order to get the best results from the treatment. In this case you can ask some pointed questions, but should avoid undermining your loved one's confidence. On the other hand, the person with cancer may need to rebel against what they are being told. I met a lady with severe cancer, Natalie, who (astonishingly) was told by her doctor that nobody got better from the degree of cancer she had. The doctor didn't know why Natalie was bothering with all the complementary therapies she was using, as her fate was sealed. Natalie's rejection of the doctor's total lack of understanding of the importance of the mind in healing stood her in good stead, and she defied her doctor by recovering! In her case, to be told that 'doctor knows best' would have been very unhelpful.

- Other relatives are able to find a balance where they are assertive and inclusive. They treat the medical staff as part of a team of equals that is led by the person with cancer. They act as a support to the cancer host, encourage them with their own approach to their treatment and healing, and generally act as a cheerleader.

The most successful way to communicate with the medical profession, as with people generally, is to be confident and assertive (but not aggressive). Don't be afraid to ask for further explanations of treatments or technical terms. If possible your loved one should do this, but you can step in to support them. Your role could be to write a list of questions or topics that the cancer host wants to cover before an appointment, and to take notes during the meeting. In fact one very positive approach would be to treat each appointment as a meeting of the 'cancer recovery project team' – although drawing up a formal agenda would probably be a step too far!

Communicating with Family and Friends

In an ideal world, a diagnosis of cancer in the family would make everyone realise what's really important. People would drop any disagreements that have been simmering, and become totally selfless. Time for a group hug, anyone?

Well, real life rarely works out quite like this. In fact people under pressure can respond amazingly. They can resolve differences, rally round and build deeper emotional connections. They can also crumble under that pressure. The chances are that the way things have been in the past will be the way they also are now.

However, there is an opportunity for *you*. Have you been holding a grudge against anyone? It's time to forgive them. Do you judge those around you and find them wanting? Stop it right now. Resolve from now on to assume that everyone is doing the best they can. If you could do better – well, that's hardly the point. They are doing the best *they* can.

In every family there are expectations built up from years past – patterns that have been created. For instance one sibling could be the responsible one, making sure all is taken care of. Another could be the 'spoilt princess'; contributing little and assuming all their needs will be met. Of course these are extreme pictures, but often our view of each other becomes set in childhood and is hard to change. We even behave differently with our families than we do in other areas of our lives.

When practical help is needed, these patterns are likely to set expectations for who will do what. It's time to question these patterns and assumptions. Just because your sister Fiona, for instance, has always been there, that doesn't mean she will be able to cope on her own supporting Mum or Dad through cancer. The demands this time will be different from how they have ever been before, so look at your expectations. Question them, and offer what support you can, without falling into the trap of 'doing everything'.

Another issue that arises with family and friends is when all their interest and attention is transferred to the cancer host. Do your siblings suddenly start calling to talk about the illness, when before you never heard from them for months? Do your friends seem to have forgotten that you're looking for a new job, or have just received a promotion, and only ask about your loved one's cancer? This is a common issue.

You may feel resentful that you have suddenly become a 'non-person'. You may tend to resist admitting this to yourself, because then you would have the guilt of your 'selfishness' to add to everything else. Well, I'd like to let you know that those feelings are natural. They're actually hard-wired into us.

I found this out when talking to one of my neighbours, Annabel, about her twins. I made the mistake of assuming that at least she didn't have to deal with sibling rivalry - because they had always both been there. "You're joking!" Annabel responded. "Since they could move their arms they have been trying to push each other off my lap so they could have me all to themselves." It's an instinct! We all want and need attention.

Don't make it harder for yourself by pretending you don't matter. Find a friend who takes an interest in *you*, not just the details of your loved one's illness, and get the attention you crave.

Communicating with Children

What to say to children about the illness of someone they care about is a thorny issue. Our instinct is to protect them from what we see as unpleasant truths. But they may be able to handle the truth better than being kept in the dark. Children are very observant. They will know if something is going on – particularly if it is affecting the emotions of those around them. Children also have vivid imaginations, and the fears they build up could be even worse than reality. If Mum and Dad snap at each other because of the emotional strain, they may imagine they don't love each other any more and could split up. So children will almost certainly cope better if they have some information.

Adapt the information for the child's age, and share it with them. Accept that they may be upset – it's only natural. Give them the chance to express how they feel about the news. This is what helps them let their feelings go naturally. Talk to them separately if you can, as different children will have different responses and different fears or concerns.

My friend Georgie found this when she told her own children about her cancer. Her 9-year-old son was very practical and clued-up about the details of the treatment – but then didn't want to be around when his Mum was ill from the effects of her chemotherapy. He was coping by keeping everything as normal as possible. In contrast, Georgie's 11-year-old daughter literally had hysterics when she heard the news. It was then important for her to see her mother regularly and get all the information on what was happening.

Just as the cancer host has to control what they can, so does the child. Let them talk to the person who has cancer, so they can see the person is still there, and still themselves. Allow them to choose how often they visit. Just make sure they have the chance to express how they feel.

They may want to be involved in the creation of a plan, like the one in the next chapter. Children can also use many of the techniques covered in this book to help them on their own journey.

You may think it would be a good idea to downplay the problem. But whatever you do, don't promise anything you can't deliver. "Of course Granny's going to get well again" may make a child feel better at the time, but what if she doesn't? Then not only do they have to deal with losing her, but also with having been 'lied to'.

It could be much fairer to let a child know that the doctors and the family are doing everything that they can to make Granny better, but no one can promise the outcome.

Communicating with Your Loved One

The way you communicated in the past with the cancer host depends on your relationship, on your respective personalities, and on the habits you have created over the years before their illness. It will be unusual if this is a relationship where you are used to talking about life, the universe and everything – simply because there aren't that many relationships like that around. If your relationship with the cancer host is like this then congratulate yourself. It will allow much easier communication.

You may find that now you have something a little more important than a trip to the supermarket to discuss with this person, it feels a little scary. The reason for this is that you're not used to it.

In my family as I was growing up, we talked about what we had done at school or what career we might like to go into. We had disagreements about emotive subjects such as abortion, but I don't remember talking about my hopes, dreams and fears with my family. We just didn't go into those topics.

What do you do if your loved one seems to shut you out – if they refuse to talk about the cancer at all? This can be really hard to cope with. It could just be the way they are coping with their situation, but that doesn't help you. You can turn to others for support, but in the end what you want is to open up the channels of communication with your loved one. It would be unrealistic to expect that you will break down those barriers in one fell swoop – and yet it is possible. The fear that comes with a diagnosis of cancer is strong enough to smash inhibitions to rubble, if you are both brave enough to admit to that fear. This may need huge courage on your part. It always seems easier to suppress the fear than talk about it, but many people report great relief from those barrier-smashing conversations.

Sometimes the resistance comes from the fact that you are used to seeing this person as strong and in charge. This may often be the case when a parent is ill, for instance. But imagine what can be gained from having your loved one share their deepest feelings with you. You may never have felt such a deep connection. I had one conversation with my mother in which she admitted her wish to die sooner rather than later. I didn't handle it well – I came out with some cliché about how it would happen when the time was right. Mum was furious; as far as she was concerned the time was right *now*, and she was fed up with waiting to be reunited with her beloved father. Well, I may not have said the right thing, but I was glad she got to express her feelings. After that talk, at least I knew how she really felt. It certainly cleared the air!

These are the conversations where you can practise your listening skills; unfortunately I hadn't learned them at this time!

From your side, what you are trying to communicate is that you love, support, respect and trust them. Even if they're not ready to talk to you, you can make sure they know this by your actions.

If you still feel more need to express yourself, why not write your loved one a letter. Tell them how much you care about them. Express your hopes and fears in writing, and they may be able to cope with this more easily.

Communicating with Yourself

As children, we are totally in touch with ourselves. We wear our heart on our sleeves and we know without a doubt what we like and don't like. My son Jason has a game he loves to play where each of us asks "What's your favourite country?" (or computer game, or animal), and everyone takes turns to answer. When was the last time someone asked you what your favourite animal is – and listened to the answer? Do you even remember? Our hopes, dreams and passions – everything that makes us ourselves – get lost over the years.

I expect that you will be having some pretty strong feelings now. Even a feeling of numbness is a feeling. The first step of communicating with yourself is to notice those feelings. This is where the listening applies to you. Recognise your hopes – and your fears. It is a good idea to set aside some time alone in order to get in touch with these feelings. You can combine this with the self-care and treats described below. If you fill your life with an endless round of looking after others then you will find the feelings are running you, and not the other way around. Handling your feelings is the Inner Journey, which is described in more detail in Chapter 6.

The other side of communicating with yourself is the message that you send to your subconscious. It is very important that this message is positive. It may be that the rest of the world is sending you a message that you don't matter, but it isn't up to the rest of the world to look after you. That's your responsibility, though of course looking after yourself can include asking others for help.

Just as 'charity begins at home', so does self-care. Start by considering the things that you enjoy – or that you used to before life got in the way. This could be uplifting music, inspirational art, a glass of wine (for pleasure, not self-medication), reading your favourite kind of book or magazine, connecting with nature, or exercise. Resolve to give yourself a treat every day. Start today. Even in the busiest life there is time to stop and look at a flower for thirty seconds. You deserve to be cared for, and who better than you to begin the process.

Choosing Your Response

In all your communications, there is one extra skill that makes things go more smoothly. This is choosing your response – also known as engaging your brain before speaking.

You can't change the circumstances that have arisen in your life, and you can't choose the things that people say to you. In both cases, though, you can choose your response.

I'm not saying it's easy. Just like your listening skills, this one may be a little under-developed. Generally we don't stop to consider our responses; we simply react. But in between the words that are spoken to you and your reply, there is a space. This is where the old advice of 'count to ten' comes into play. The trick is to notice the space – and make it bigger. If you can feel love or empathy for the person you are communicating with, then you can fill the gap with that feeling, and the response you choose will come from that love.

In order to notice the gap and choose your response, you will need concentration and focus. If you are thinking about everything else that needs to be done – the laundry, cleaning or your other worries – that concentration will be missing. In coaching we call this 'getting present with the client', and it is like switching from Level I to

Level II listening.

If you are truly present in the communication that is happening now, not dancing off into the past or the future, then you can choose your response. By listening at Level II or III, and by responding rather than reacting, you are doing all in your power to deepen every communication that you have.

Not every conversation will go well, for you have no control over the other person, or their emotions. At least you will know that you put your best into communicating with them.

Communicating without Words

Most of this chapter so far has been about how we communicate with words, though the levels of listening did touch on a deeper level.

Have you ever had a conversation with someone where their actions didn't match up with what they said? They claim to care about you, but you find it hard to believe them, for instance. I well remember talking to my ex about splitting up. He wanted us to stay together and talked a lot about how great our relationship was. The trouble was that as time went by, there was no change in his behaviour. We never spoke about the issue again until the time I left him. The message I received from him, loud and clear, was that our relationship wasn't as important as his convenience, even though his words said something different.

There are lots of ways that we communicate without words.

We do it by touch (or lack of it), by what we do for someone, through our eyes and our tone of voice. Don't underestimate the importance of these kinds of communication.

Premature babies fare better if they are stroked for even a small amount of time each day. At the other end of the scale, one problem for many in their later years is the fact that no-one ever touches them other than in a clinical way to administer some medical procedure. This is one of the reasons that massage (or even a manicure) is so beneficial.

Touch is very important in your communications, too. In this you need to be guided by the person themselves as to the kinds of touch they are comfortable with. The cancer host may also have reactions that make touch difficult for them.

As my mother became more ill, she was unable to tolerate touch very well. Don't take it personally if it is this way for your loved one. If they don't tell you in words, you will be able to know from their body language if something is making them uncomfortable.

Giving someone your undivided attention also shows how important they are to you. Small loving gestures or gifts might also be suitable, so long as they don't make the recipient feel that you are treating them as incapable.

One of the deepest methods of communication we have, with our life partners, is sex. This is why it is such a powerful part of a loving relationship. At its best, in a loving relationship, sex goes beyond words and allows you to feel as one with your partner. If your partner is the one who has cancer, you may assume that sex has to go, but don't leap to conclusions. There will probably be times when they don't feel able, but withdrawing from intimacy may also be the last thing they want. It could be vital for your partner to feel they are still attractive to you. Once again, you will have to take your cue from them.

ACTION STEP

In order to practise your communication skills, aim to find out three things you didn't know about other people every day. This could be three things about the same person, or one thing about three separate people. If this is too easy, raise the bar and aim for ten.

Even if you don't manage to speak to anyone that day, you can think over past conversations and have a realisation you never had before. You might find out that your friend doesn't eat cheese, that the lady at the shop checkout doesn't get off work until 8 pm, or that your life partner was unhappy at school. Anything is possible!

4

PLANNING FOR A MORE SUCCESSFUL JOURNEY

How do you approach a trip you are intending to take? Do you just set off and hope for the best? Or are you more like my father, who plans his walking trips much like a military campaign? Months of obtaining bus timetables, maps and leaflets take place before he sets off.

You may be wondering what this has to do with your loved one's cancer, as your journey has already started without any planning. Even if it's not your natural style, though, there is a benefit of taking some time now to plan as much as you can. If you are like my father, this may come naturally, if not then at least you have a good reason to learn.

Successful Journeys Take Planning

I confess that I'm a natural planner – there, I've admitted it. I guess it comes from my Dad. I feel uncomfortable making a journey without having done at least some research. My experience has been that it usually saves time, and makes everything go more smoothly.

I suppose I'm a believer in the old saying, "He who fails to plan, plans to fail." The point of planning is to get to know a little of the terrain ahead. In coaching we call it a 'meta-view' – rising up from where you are now to look at the bigger picture. You could think of it as a bird's eye view. Once you have that view, you are more prepared to travel through that terrain, and to know what resources you may need.

This planning is something positive you can do to assist your loved one and yourself to get through this challenge. It is possible that the cancer host can only see the next rock on the path ahead. At times this may be their job – to focus only on the current challenge. You, however, are able to take a step back and see that 'this, too, will pass'.

Plan Even Though the Journey has Already Started

Unlike most journeys, you have not had the opportunity to plan before it began. This is one of the reasons why your fear and uncertainty is so great. You are not in control – and that is an understatement! At this point you can only accept that you couldn't plan before you knew there was a journey to take. It's not too late to make a difference, though.

If you were leading a community fleeing from a natural

disaster, you would probably send out scouting parties ahead. They would report back on what they found, such as hazards in the path ahead, and you could choose the route for the group in view of that. Planning on the move can still make a difference to how successful your journey will be.

Create a Cancer Success Plan

At last, a way to wrest some control from the jaws of uncertainty - create a Cancer Success Plan. This grand-sounding document can be as simple or as fancy as you like. It can be something you create with the person who has cancer, or just for your own use. It can be anything from a computer file to an enormous binder stuffed with vast reams of information.

In other words, you get to choose. You are in complete control of this, at least. It is likely that you won't have all the information at the beginning, but creating the plan gives you somewhere to put information as you get it.

What should you put in this marvellous resource you are going to create? Well, it will be as individual as you, but here are some suggestions for sections you may want to include:

- *What success is to you*
  This is particularly important (see **Defining Success In Your Cancer Journey**, below). *Don't skip this section.*
- *Where you are now*
  What the current situation is with your loved one's health, your home life, your stress levels and anything else that is relevant.

- *Taking care of yourself*

  A list of things and activities to make you feel good, or lower your stress level.

- *Information on specific cancer*

  You will probably want to include specific information about the type of cancer your loved one has (see **Getting Hold of Information**, below).

- *Treatment plan and record*

  What has been suggested, what the cancer host has agreed to. What treatments they have been given and what effect those have had.

- *Support groups and therapies*

  Information you gather about support groups, organisations and complementary therapies for yourself as well as your loved one. You may want to include our website, www.familiesfacingcancer.org.

- *Positive activities to share*

  Don't forget to make time to do something fun together. Make it realistic for your loved one, but enough fun to be worthwhile.

- *Help that has been offered*

  When friends and family offer to help, get a specific commitment and make a record of it.

- *Contingency*

  These are resources you may never need, but may call on if necessary. (See **Contingency planning**, below and also Chapter 7, When The Going Gets Tough.)

There is one other thing I think would be immensely useful in your plan, and it refers back to **Losing the Victim Label** in Chapter 2.

In order to assist you in thinking of your loved one as a whole and healthy person, I suggest you include a photograph of them. Choose one that you feel shows their best qualities: your favourite photograph of them. You may think that this will only remind you of what has currently been lost, but I maintain that it is not lost. That is still the person they are. Every time you look at the picture, let go of any regret you feel and tell yourself that this is still the person you love.

Next, let's expand on some of the sections of your plan which need a little more explanation.

Defining 'Success' in Your Cancer Journey

The reason I insisted that you don't skip this section is because I think you may be tempted to do exactly that – but don't.

Your first reaction may be that of course you know what success means – it means your loved one gets better! There are two problems with this as a definition of success in the journey:

1. It's not specific enough.

    The Director of Blythe House Hospice told me that they consider there are many different possible outcomes to cancer, not simply whether the person lives or dies. For instance the cancer could go into remission, but the person's family relationships could have been destroyed in the process. That wouldn't be such a great success.

2.   It is outside your control.

If the *only* definition of success you have depends on factors that are totally outside your control, you are left at the mercy of the fates. Success or failure depends not on you, but on the cancer host and how their disease progresses. There is little you can do to make a difference.

All right, so 'my loved one gets better' is not a definition of success that works here, though you may of course want to describe your desire for that outcome as part of this section. You could also include in your definition of success that the cancer host feels as little distress as possible.

The wishes of the person with cancer may also affect the definition of success. You should know by now whether they want to fight, or feel they are at the whim of fate. Often with a first diagnosis of cancer the reaction of the person is a fierce "I'm not ready to die". But this is not always the case – and that may alter what success means for both of you.

One other way to define success is to look at your whole life using the life-coaching tool The Wheel of Life (see diagram below; you can download a printable version from our website). Traditionally you would look at where you are on each section of the wheel, mark a score on the chart, and set a goal for each area. I'm suggesting a slightly different use. If you look at each section, it relates to an area of your life. Write down what the current situation is for you in that area of your life, and how your loved one's cancer affects that area. This will mean you have also covered the **Where you are now** section in your plan, to some extent. Then define what success means in that area taking into account your current situation.

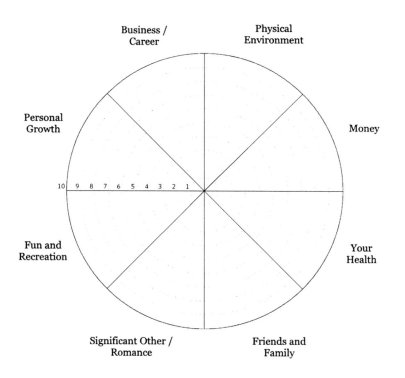

Wheel of Life Chart

Here is an example. In the area of Family and Friends, you have a tricky relationship with one of your siblings. This has been made worse by one of your parents being diagnosed with cancer. Success in this area, then, might be to use the situation to 'make up with' that person and improve your relationship with them.

Success in the area of Business/Career, however, might be to keep your job in spite of the pressures on you, or it could be to cut your hours in order to lessen that pressure.

Whatever you write in this section, don't assume that it is set in stone. You are writing a plan, not a contract. You can and will alter it as time goes by.

One thing that is certain is that you will not be entirely the same person at the end of your journey with another's cancer (that does not have to be a bad thing, by the way). This means that your vision of what success means may also change along the way.

Getting Hold of Information

There are many different ways to find information for your plan.

Before you start, consider how much information you want or need. Too much negative information could be depressing and create an unhelpful expectation for you. I sometimes think it is amazing that anyone's health improves by taking prescription drugs as reading the list of potential side effects is so frightening!

Of course you want to know what is involved in the exact type of cancer that your loved one is dealing with. All cancers are as individual as their hosts, but the broad group into which this cancer falls will tell you something about what to expect. I would say, though, that there is a huge range of possible outcomes for any cancer. Whereabouts on the scale your friend or relative will be depends on many factors, not least their own mind-set.

So where do you go to find out more information? The first place is information provided by the medical team treating the cancer host. The team may have provided leaflets for them to read about the type of cancer they have, or any proposed treatments. You can also contact cancer charities such as Macmillan or Cancer*Care*, who will do their best to inform you.

Another source of information is local groups and organisations. These could include hospices or support groups. You may want to buy books to read which could give you hope or information, or borrow them from your local library. The book that resonates most with me on cancer and its treatment is *The Bristol Approach to Living with Cancer* produced by Penny Brohn Cancer Care.

In our modern world, there is also a vast amount of information on the internet. It is important when finding information in this way to consider the source. Does the advice given seem impartial, or does it only exist to sell a high-priced 'cure'? By all means don't discount anything, but most good information will be backed up by more than one reputable source. You could find a lot of conflicting information, and if you can't decide what to believe you may want to trust your gut feel. Your intuition is very wise and you should listen to it.

If you want help in finding sources of information you can visit the resources section of our website, www.familiesfacingcancer.org. Please also let us know of any information sources that have been particularly helpful to you, so that we can share them with others.

Taking the Time to Find Your Own Truth

It would be easy in this planning phase to become very focused on the needs of the cancer host, and what the outcome will be for them. This is a reminder that it is your planning. Even if you are creating a plan together, it is vital that you take the time to look at your own hopes and fears. How does their cancer affect you? What would success be in terms of learning and growing from this challenge?

It may feel self-indulgent to spend this time on yourself, but it's not. This is the only life you have right now, and you must live through this situation. You cannot afford to set your own feelings aside.

Taking Direction from Your Loved One

Whilst you are considering your own needs, hopes and dreams, you will have to temper this by considering the desires of the cancer host. The way people react to having cancer varies, and the situation in which people find themselves at the time may make an enormous difference.

When my mother was diagnosed with secondary brain tumours, we all wanted her to defy medical logic and get better. Her point of view was that she was not very attached to being alive, even though we were attached to her being here. Perhaps if her job had been less stressful, or her father had still been alive, she might have felt differently. But she didn't. Overcoming enormous medical odds takes a special kind of determination, which Mum didn't have. We could have listened better, and taken our definitions of success from what worked for her.

Of course, your relationship and the conversations you have can make a lot of difference to how your loved one feels. If they know you believe in seeing them restored to health, it could give them the confidence they need to fight. Encourage your loved one to talk about both their hopes and their fears. Find out how they feel about the future.

Many people with cancer find a deep desire to live (such as having young children and being determined to be around for them), and go on to recover seemingly by sheer force of will.

The communication skills you learned in the last chapter will be put to good use here. It is important to open the channels of communication now. However good they have been in the past you are going to need them now more than ever.

Be Responsible for Your Journey, Not Theirs

Taking direction from your loved one in their cancer journey is also a matter of separation. Your love and support may contribute to the outcome of their cancer, but you can't take the journey for them. You can never feel exactly what they feel.

Have you ever shared something that happened with someone else, only to have them reply "Oh, I know exactly how you feel" and launch into a description of something that happened to them? How did you react to that? Did you feel understood and supported, or did you think "They really have no idea what I'm going through"?

You *don't* know exactly what the cancer host is going through – even if you've had cancer yourself. You're not the same person they are, however connected to them you feel. The good news is you don't need to understand; just listen to what they tell you and accept it is true for them. It's not your job to take this journey for your loved one;

they are quite capable of doing it for themselves. Not only that, you owe it to them to allow them the journey.

When a child is learning to do something new, like tie their shoelaces, at the beginning we tell them at every step what to do next. At some stage, though, we have to let them try it out for themselves. Otherwise they will not become independent and strong.

Even if the cancer host is a child, you must allow them control over their own illness – their own journey. They can understand what is happening to them and make decisions about their own treatment, if they have support in doing so. You have enough to think about being responsible for your own journey and your own learning.

Contingency Planning

I have already touched on facing up to the thought that the eventual outcome of your loved one's cancer could be death. You don't have to like that option – I would probably be worried if you did at the beginning. But you must face this possibility. Even as you begin your journey with another's cancer, I'm asking you to consider what will happen if things get worse. You will find much more about this in Chapter 7.

This section of your plan could contain details of what you know about the cancer host's will, or their wishes should they die. Now I'm not suggesting you sit down and raise the topic on day one. Just allow them to talk about these things as you share your hopes and fears with them. It may be important for them to do so, rather than bottling up these thoughts.

This section of your plan may also contain resources that you don't need now, but could call on if the need arises. This could include your local hospice or respite centre. This brings us on to the kind of resources you want to include in the plan, and how to find out about them.

Adding Resources to Your Plan

What kind of resources can help you in your journey? I think these break down into two kinds of resource.

One kind is local resources that you can make use of in person. The other is more distant or general resources you use over the telephone or internet.

I will look at how these resources can be of help to you in more detail in the following two chapters, but for now here are some ideas of the resources that can help you. Your aim is to build up a list of contact details or notes about these resources, so that you can make use of them as your journey progresses.

1.   **Local resources**

   - *Support groups*
     Local support groups exist for both cancer hosts and carers. You can probably find out about them from your doctor, either locally or at the hospital where your loved one is being treated.

   - *Hospices and specialist centres*
     Local hospices are a wonderful resource, and contrary to popular myth, no one needs to be dying in order to use

them. They may have criteria to decide who can make use of their services, as there are great demands on their resources. Check to see what those criteria are. Then add those details to your resource list together with the services that the hospice offers. Charities such as Macmillan in the UK also have support centres.

- *Therapists*

   There are many complementary therapies that can be of great help to both you and the cancer host. There is more detail about the ways these can help in the next two chapters, and on our website. You may be able to find details of them through local directories, or by recommendation from friends.

- *Other Interest Groups*

   Not every resource needs to be specific to dealing with cancer. Joining a book group or model railway society may be just the antidote you need. Exercise can be particularly supportive of your own health and well being, so you may want to search out exercise classes or walking groups.

2. General resources

- *Books and e-books*

   Of course, this book is a wonderful resource (I hope!), but you may have many other books recommended to you. If you note down the book name and author when you hear of it, you will be able to get hold of it when it will be most helpful.

- *Chat rooms*

  There are many Internet groups devoted to the subject of cancer, and they can be a source of immense support. For instance, Macmillan have their Share group which you can access from anywhere in the world through their website. It is filled with supportive people, many of whom have taken, or are taking, a journey similar to yours. We also have forums at www.familiesfacingcancer.org, so why not stop by and share the highs and lows of your journey.

- *Telephone helplines*

  There may be times when you want to ask a question and there is no one on hand to give you that specific information. Telephone helplines run by cancer charities and hospices can be helpful at these times. Whether it is just someone to offload to, or a specific question about your loved one's treatment, they may be able to set your mind at rest.

- *Coaches, and counsellors*

  Both life coaching and counselling can take place over the telephone. If you would like more specific one-to-one support from someone who gets to know you and your situation, consider adding a professional life coach or counsellor to your support team.

You can find contact details for many of these resources at our website www.familiesfacingcancer.org. You can also help us to build up our resource list by giving us details of resources you have used.

Adding Energy

You may wonder what energy has to do with your Plan, but of course I don't mean electricity. I mean the mental and emotional feel of your plan.

Imagine for instance if it was called a Cancer Survival Plan. How would that be different from your Cancer Success Plan? What changes would you make to the contents? A Cancer Attack Plan would be a different thing again. The words we use make a big difference to the energy with which we live our lives. They also change the results that we see. T. Harv Eker (one of my personal development teachers) taught me that "What I Focus on Expands", and this is one reason for carefully choosing words. If your plan had an 'Emergency' section, then you would be focusing on emergencies. Using the word 'Contingency' sounds like something that's not very likely – and so has better energy.

You may think that I am contradicting myself, because I've told you to look at the worst possible scenario – that of your loved one dying. But even a death can be positive or negative, depending on the circumstances and how you look at them. You can visit the website **www.hospiceoftheheart.org** where you can find information on gentle dying, i.e. creating a 'good death'. Dealing with these darkest fears allows you to let them go and put your focus on the positive side where it belongs.

Other ways to add positive energy include the photograph I suggested, showing the cancer host as healthy and happy. You could also add a picture of the two of you together.

Your Cancer Success Plan should be a document you enjoy

picking up. You could decorate it with your own drawings, beautiful pictures you have printed or cut out of magazines, cartoons or jokes. You might want a section for inspirational poems or quotes you come across. You could use a pretty notebook for your plan. Writing headings (or everything!) in colour adds a brighter feel, and will engage you if you are a kinaesthetic type of person. (This is you if you are more interested in how things feel than how they look.)

The section on **Taking care of yourself** will put a positive slant on the plan. You should put this near the beginning, as you are important, not an afterthought. Lots of good energy can go into the section on **Positive activities to share**. Try to make some of these activities little things you can do on a day-to-day basis, like finding jokes to share with each other. Then put in some longer-term plans, such as a visit to somewhere you always meant to go. This gives you and the cancer host the fun and distraction of planning.

Letting Go of Attachment

Now you have your Plan – or at least the beginning of it. So you know what's going to happen and how things will go in the future, right? Wrong! If I've learned one thing about life, it's that nothing is predictable.

I've made many changes in my life: getting divorced; moving from one area of the UK to another; having my children. These were changes I chose myself. There are many other changes I had no control over. My mother's illness, for instance. I learned as time went by to go with the flow. I ask myself what is inside my circle of influence. I control what I can, and go along with the way things turn out for the rest.

I once took a trip with my best friend, who was living in Seattle, to Vancouver. We visited Vancouver Island for the day, then sailed to the mainland. The plan was to find somewhere to stay on the Olympic Peninsula, and then visit the Hoh Rainforest the next day. I would have preferred to book a place to stay, but my friend wouldn't have it – and it turned out there wasn't a room to be had in town. As we'd arrived off the ferry at 9 pm, this left us with few options, so we started driving. Sooner or later, we thought, we would find somewhere to stay. Well, it wasn't to be, and we drove back to Seattle through the night. The journey didn't go according to plan. I still haven't visited the Hoh Rainforest, but I remember that night. I remember taking turns to drive, country and western music on the radio, and the comradeship of the road trip. It wasn't the journey we had in mind, but it's a journey I recall clearly 20 years later.

However your journey turns out, the key is to make the most of it along the way.

This is another form of energy for your plan. If you *need* your loved one to get better, then you will be operating from the energy of fear. If you can be at peace with the outcome, whatever it may be, you will be able to stay more positive throughout. Enjoy the times you have together, whether it be two weeks or twenty years.

ACTION STEP

No prizes for this one. Start your Cancer Success Plan! If you've done that already, then add what you can. Don't let the lack of a folder or book delay you. Start today. Find a piece of paper or the back of an envelope and write the words Cancer Success Plan. If you don't have a pen, borrow one from a neighbour. No excuses. Now, you're on the journey.

"A good plan today is better than a perfect plan tomorrow!"

5

THE OUTER JOURNEY – PRACTICAL CONSIDERATIONS

Your journey has already started. You have done your best to adjust to that. You are practising and expanding your communication skills. You have planned as much as you can at this stage. Now there is nothing left between you and reality. It's time to look at some issues that may come up during your journey. How will you handle them? What will make your journey go more smoothly?

What to Expect During Treatment

One feature of cancer that is different from many other diseases is the effect of the treatment that is designed to cure the person receiving it. In most illnesses, treatments work on the basis of suppressing symptoms, or supporting the person's body in working as well as it can. Cancer treatment is different. Lou Reed described it well in a song entitled *The Sword of Damocles*. It contains the line "To cure you they must kill you" – a spot-on description.

Surgery may be used to remove a tumour, but will almost always be followed up with either chemotherapy or radiotherapy. The job of both these treatments is to destroy any remaining cancer cells. The trouble is that they are not very targeted. They just kill cells. As the cancer cells are dividing faster than normal, they are more likely to die, but other cells will also be affected.

Scientists are working on better, targeted and more effective treatments, but what I have described is still the approach for most cancers – if indeed any curative treatment can be offered. Adam Wishart's book *One In Three: a son's journey into the science and history of cancer* covers how these treatments developed and what is hoped for the future.

The problem is that our bodies are not a collection of unrelated parts. They are an incredibly complex integrated system, and science has barely scraped the surface of understanding that system. What affects one part of the system affects it all, and you will see the results of this.

What this means to you is that under conventional cancer treatments, the person you know is likely to get worse before they get better. My mother-in-law, May, seemed perfectly well when she was diagnosed with breast cancer. She was young for her years, active and still working part time at the age of 72. She was then faced with surgery, exercises to mobilise her arm and rounds of chemotherapy which brought on nausea, tiredness and loss of her hair. On the face of things, it was the *treatment* that made her ill, and from which she needed to recover.

What can you expect for your loved one? The hospital will probably give some information to the cancer host on the possible 'side effects' of the treatment they are offered. They may not want too much of this information, so it may be a good idea for you to read it. There could be helpful suggestions for dealing with specific problems. There is a vast quantity of information in *The Chemotherapy and Radiation Therapy Survival Guide* by Judith McKay and Nancee Hirano. This is a book I turned to for information during May's treatment. You could include the information you find in your Cancer Success Plan.

Common physical responses to treatment include extreme tiredness, nausea, loss of appetite, hair loss from chemotherapy, skin reactions, plus feeling very cold and a change of physical features due to water retention. Responses may also occur after treatments which are not intended to be curative but palliative (managing symptoms), such as with the steroids my mother was given.

Adults undergoing cancer treatment may appear to age rapidly, but this could be a temporary response to the treatment. It can be hard to watch someone you love decline physically, so try to keep 'the real them' in your mind using the picture from your Plan. There will also be emotional responses to treatment. Tiredness may cause irritability, for instance. Fear of both the disease and the treatment may come out as anger towards those around them. If your loved one's personality seems to change, don't take it personally. It could be related either to the disease or to the treatment. Try to let any aggression slide off you, or release the emotions it provokes in you using the techniques described in the next chapter, The Inner Journey.

There may be ways to lessen the unwanted effects of treatment, and you may want to investigate whether any of those are suitable for your loved one (as long as they are happy for you to do this). One way would be to consult Penny Brohn Cancer Care, or read their book *The Bristol Approach to Living with Cancer*. Other holistic support centres may help with this issue.

My mother-in-law had homeopathic support during her treatment, and the nurses were amazed at the speed of her recovery from surgery. Visualisation can also be helpful in allowing the cancer host to gain more benefit from their treatment with less adverse effects. There may be someone locally who could support your loved one in learning these techniques before their treatment. NLP practitioners work with the mind and visualisation and so may be able to help in this way.

What if They Refuse Treatment?

It is not unusual for a person diagnosed with cancer to refuse conventional treatment entirely. If you consider what I said about the ferocity of those treatments, you can hardly blame them. Your loved one may have heard amazing tales of people who recovered from cancer with no conventional treatment whatsoever. The story of Cathy Goodman is featured in the book and film *The Secret*, and she literally thought herself well. It may be that your friend or relative could also do this. It is their decision to make.

I would sound a small note of caution, however. I totally believe in the body's ability to heal itself, even in extreme situations.

However, I know that it can take time. It also takes a very positive outlook on life and, often, radical dietary shifts.

Cancers come in many different forms. Some are slow-growing, and may give plenty of time for self-healing. Others are more aggressive, and time for treatment is of the essence.

If the cancer host is reluctant to embark on a difficult course of treatment, don't get mad at them. Whatever you do, don't try to force them into taking the treatment against their will. It is a rare case where there isn't even a day available for reflection, so take some time. Talk through the pros and cons with your loved one. What are they afraid of? What is the likely progress of the cancer if they leave conventional treatment out for now? How could they mix complementary approaches with the conventional treatment being offered? Could conventional treatment be safely delayed for a while to allow the cancer host to try other approaches? Decisions are not usually black and white. There is almost always a third option, if you take the time to look.

Natalie, whom I mentioned in Chapter 3, was reluctant to undergo medical treatments, and wanted to rely on alternative healing. After all, her doctor had told her she was going to die, so she saw little point in rounds of tough chemotherapy. She had the right to make that choice, but her family *asked* her to take the treatment. They supported her in adding the dietary changes and healing treatments she desired to the regime suggested by the hospital. This is the route she finally chose, honouring her husband's and children's wishes. When we last spoke she was, happily, free from cancer.

Taking on More of The Load

Your loved one will be undergoing either conventional treatment or a self-help regime they have devised themselves (or a combination, of course). Whichever route they are taking, it's likely that they won't be able to continue with all the activities they did before. This may vary from time to time depending on treatment or how well they feel. At some point, though, someone else is going to have to shoulder more of the load. Some partners of people who have cancer find that they have become full-time carers. Many adult children find they have to help out their parents at a time when their own lives may be busy and full of stress.

Before you rush in like Wonder Woman or Superman, taking on your loved one's duties, stop for a moment. How do you know what they need you to do? How do you know they're not doing just fine without you? Have you checked, or are you making assumptions?

My mother-in-law managed well through her cancer treatment. I'm not saying she had it easy, and she did stay with her nephew for a short time after her surgery. She found, though, that she preferred to be at home alone after the chemotherapy. If she had to feel ill, she would rather be on her own. After each dose, she would be back at work within days. I wanted to go and stay with her while she was having the treatment, so that I could help, but she wouldn't have it. I realise now that having me fussing around would have driven her mad. Doing it her way, she could be herself, and get back to normal as soon as possible.

Not everyone copes so well, of course. The cancer host may not be able to keep up with their previous level of activity. Certainly my mother was unable to carry on looking after the house as she became more ill, and that did cause her some distress. Even though my father in particular took on some of her usual tasks, they weren't done to her satisfaction. These were tasks such as the housework and cooking, but better to try than to starve was Dad's opinion. Whilst we saw her distress, there seemed no way to relieve it. Looking back, I'm not sure the house was ever as clean and tidy as she would have liked it – especially when all four children were still living there!

So in fact this wasn't really something new, and all the cleaning in the world would not have made her well. I dread to think what she would have said about the state my house got into while I was writing this book – but then she often despaired of me!

When you are considering taking on tasks for the cancer host, run through these questions before you do so:

1. Could this person still complete the task to their own satisfaction? If so, is it adversely affecting their health for them to do so, or is it benefiting them?
2. Does this task have to be done, or is it being continued out of habit? What would happen if it were just omitted for a while?
3. What will be gained from this task being done?
4. Does it have to be me that takes on the task? Is there someone more suited, or could outside help be brought in (and paid for if necessary)?
5. If I take on this task, what other task will I drop? Does this other task I will omit give less benefit than the task I'm taking on?

The last question is especially important. Unless you are

bored and have spare time, then taking on new tasks will mean that something else suffers – either it will go, or you won't do it as well. You need to weigh up the benefits. Consider if you spent less time with your children in order to go and clean your mother's house, for example, as I described above. Yes, you might ease her distress a little, but her house will be dirty again next week. That time with your children can never be regained.

My father felt that time spent talking to my mother, reading the Bible together and making the most of the time they had, was of more value to both of them than a clean house.

Being at a Distance

The usual image of a carer or supporter is of someone close to the person who is ill, maybe living with them or possibly close by. In our world today, though, we don't always live close to our families. We can be separated by hundreds of miles, or even live at the other side of the world. How do you cope, knowing that your loved one is ill but you're not there? What practical considerations are going to come up as a result?

First of all, don't discount the support you can offer just because you are far away. Of course you will visit if you are able, but you can also support on the telephone or via email. You are still in a position to do a lot.

So what *can* you do to handle the issue of being far away?

- Go to visit the person if it is at all possible, as soon as you can manage after they are diagnosed – as long as this is something they want. You will be able to communicate with them much better face to face, and it will be reassuring for you to know you have been to see them.

- If you do visit, find a way not to add to their workload. This can be difficult with some people, especially women who are legends in their own kitchens. Imagine if the whole family descends, though. They could end up wearing themselves out catering for everyone. It's not going to do any favours for their health. Find another way if you can without treating the cancer host as incapable. This could be as simple as suggesting you go out for a meal, or offering to fetch a takeaway.

- If the cancer host does not want you to visit or you can't do so, find out the best way to communicate with them. Do they want to talk on the phone, or chat by email? Bear in mind that you're not the only person who wants to talk to them, so try to be patient.

- Ask them what you can do to help, and make some suggestions. Would they like you to send them jokes and cartoons? Do they need to know they can ring you to unload when they're feeling down? Knowing what you can do to help will lessen the feeling of frustration from being far away.

- Make sure you know who is there to help. If you don't live close by, then find out who is there. Are there other relatives who will go to hospital appointments with the cancer host? Or maybe they have close friends who will help in some way. There may also be local cancer support organisations. If you know who is there, it may help to set your mind at rest.

Managing Tiredness

One issue that you are likely to face is that of tiredness, sometimes made worse by insomnia. I can't underestimate the effect of this; chronic tiredness can have a severe effect on your health, your work and your relationships. Some of the weariness you feel will be to do with trying to (or having to) do more, particularly if you are caring for someone who is very ill. You can avoid at least some of this if you are careful about what you take on. Some tiredness may be unavoidable, especially for those who live with the cancer host. You may have disturbed sleep for a long time if you are needed in the night to help your loved one. Parents of young children often know all too well the toll this can take.

You can seem to get used to an irregular sleep pattern. Usually, though, when you are able to return to normal you realise the effect the disturbance was having in terms of how you felt during the day, and your level of concentration. If you are struggling, plan ahead to get some times when you can sleep properly. Getting extra sleep might involve someone coming in to help you with the caring (either relatives or nurses). On the other hand you could use respite care at a hospice for the cancer host in order to give you a break.

You can manage physical tiredness by being realistic about what you can do in the time you have – and not doing more than that.

You might think that being tired will mean you find it easy to get to sleep when you get the chance, but for some people insomnia becomes a real issue. This is mainly due to stress, and can attack you at either end of the night. Some people have great difficulty getting to sleep, and others wake early in the morning with their brain whirring in a high gear. This can become a vicious circle as you start to worry that you're not getting enough sleep, which makes your mind even more active.

The first way to tackle insomnia is to deal with any physical causes. These include being too active in the evening with no time to wind down; for some people an excess of caffeine; or not having a calm space in which to sleep. Try to create a bedtime routine that helps you fall asleep, if that is where your problem lies. What has helped you sleep well in the past?

Once the physical issues are dealt with, you are left with the mental and emotional. First and foremost, don't try to fight insomnia. On the (admittedly rare) occasions that I have had trouble sleeping, I just get up and read a book for a while. When I feel tired enough, I then go back to sleep.

Viktor Frankl, in his book *Man's Search For Meaning*, explains that trying too hard can prevent us being able to achieve what we want. His suggestion would be to try to stay awake. You might want to start meditating. In my experience, if you decide you want to meditate for half an hour, it will be very hard to stay awake for that time if your body is in need of sleep. If you do stay awake, you will have gained a lot of benefit from the meditation.

If you follow the journey in the next chapter then you will also deal with many of the thoughts and emotions that could be keeping you awake. A large part of tiredness can be caused by the emotional stress of the situation, and you will find techniques there to help you relieve this stress.

You can also use complementary therapies to relieve stress, as described below in **Maintaining Energy through Complementary**

Therapies. Unresolved issues and worry are the major cause of unwanted early morning wakefulness. If this is a problem in your life, you need to work on your Inner Journey, which I cover in the next chapter. Finally, why not visit our website to share resources that have helped you or others deal with tiredness or insomnia.

Making Space for Yourself

When the focus is so firmly on someone else, you can feel as though you are becoming a non-person. I described this in Chapter 3 under **Communicating with Family and Friends**. It's almost as if you were being squeezed out of existence. You can counteract this effect, but in order to do so you will first have to accept that you have the right to some time and space to yourself.

Creating a literal, physical space for yourself could be especially important if you live with the person who has cancer. In this case it can seem difficult to escape the pressure, when you are together much of the time. See if there is a corner of your home that can become a retreat for you. If you are starting to meditate, this could be a good time to set up a quiet corner in a spare room if you have one. You could set aside a comfy chair where you intend to write in your journal. Men (and even some women) have often retreated to the garden shed to potter. Even the bathroom could become an oasis of calm where you can escape for half an hour if you add a few candles. It doesn't matter what the space is, so long as it is yours. You should feel more peaceful there, and being there will remind you that you are taking time for yourself. If there really isn't a single corner of your home that will do, perhaps you can gain the same benefits from a local park, or the seafront.

Making space for you also means mental space. If you have hobbies or interests, think very carefully before giving them up. I watched a programme on television about people whose hobby was racing homing pigeons. One of the people featured was a man whose wife had Alzheimer's disease, and needed a lot of care. At one point in the programme he said "I suppose I should give up my pigeons, but they keep me sane." It really can be as necessary as that to keep up your hobbies. It could make the difference between your coping with the situation and falling apart. Even if you don't feel your own stresses are as extreme as this man's, there is a great benefit to having something else to think about for a while.

What if you don't have any hobbies? Simple – just start one. Either something you used to do but gave up, or an interest you've been meaning to pursue and not found the time. Trust me, it will be worth taking the time now to do this.

Maintaining Energy through Complementary Therapies

If you are under pressure, and you have to keep going, you need a support team. It's no good ploughing on and ignoring your own needs, then buckling under the strain. You may think that only the cancer host will benefit from complementary therapies. Far from it. Therapies are not just for dealing with illness; they have a lot to offer in maintaining your body and your energy at this time of stress.

It's not the job of this book to cover how complementary therapies benefit those with cancer – I am focusing on how to help you. If you do want to learn more about this, you could read the book I referred to before – *The Bristol Approach to Living with Cancer* or Deepak Chopra's *Quantum Healing*. Do remember, though, that your loved one's recovery is their responsibility – it is not up to you to make decisions for them, unless they are incapable of doing so.

Anyway, back to you. Here is a selection of methods you could use to maintain your energy levels.

- **Massage**. Whilst we often think of massage as a method of relaxation, or for treating physical problems, it can be of use in many situations. A good massage therapist can tailor a treatment to be either relaxing or energising. In fact there are many therapists who specialise in workplace massage – where total relaxation is definitely not wanted. So a massage can deliver whatever you need at the time, quite apart from being a pleasant form of touch.

- **Acupuncture**. Whilst it is often used for physical ailments, acupuncture works on energy pathways in the body. Any imbalances caused by this stressful situation can be resolved, before any symptoms become apparent.

- **Reiki or Crystal Healing**. These therapies work directly on your energy, either through the therapist's hands or using crystals. I personally find both of them extremely relaxing and effective. They certainly give you time to yourself, and allow your body to find its own balance.

- **Reflexology**. This is again a therapy that people tend to turn to for physical ailments, but is equally effective for stress relief. I used it during my first pregnancy, more to promote a general sense of well being than to resolve any specific issue.

- **Homeopathy**. A homeopath will consider everything about their client, including their emotional state and the stress that they are feeling. In fact there are specific remedies that are particularly indicated when dealing with shock or trauma. Homeopathy also has the benefit that some practitioners consult over the telephone, so this could be more convenient for you if you are busy. The aim would be to boost both your physical and emotional resilience to the current situation.

Keep on Exercising

I'm sure you already know all the physical reasons why exercise is a good thing. Did you also know that it is an excellent stress reliever? There are two main reasons for this, which may well be connected. Firstly, exercising helps your brain switch off. Even repetitive exercise, which you would imagine would give you more time to think, lulls the mind into getting a bit quieter. I don't know why this happens, but I do know it's a good thing! Secondly, when you exercise your body produces feel-good substances called endorphins. These are the body's natural high, without any of the unwanted effects of other substances we use to give us a lift. Exercise also gives you more energy, as your body strengthens in response to how much you use it. So don't give up lightly any exercise you do already.

If you aren't exercising at the moment, you could add some in – starting slowly, of course. You will have to be practical about the time you have available, I know. Whatever exercise works for you is good; even 10 minutes of toning up your muscles makes a difference.

You could learn Callanetics, which is a form of exercise you can do easily at home.

If you have a regular job, you may be able to fit exercise into your lunch hour, or before or after work. This could overcome the lethargy that often takes over when we have to go out specially to exercise.

If resistance is keeping you from getting going, you could try the "Well, I'll just" approach. Never heard of it? Say you're planning to go for a run, or a swim, but you just feel too tired to exercise today. Then you say to yourself "Well, I'll just put my running gear on", or "Well, I'll just drive to the swimming pool". This gets you out of your chair, without committing you to anything much. Naturally, once you've got the gear on, or you're sitting outside the pool, you've beaten the resistance already. It would seem silly not to go on and do the exercise! Of course, it does help if you've chosen a form of exercise you enjoy, because then you might even look forward to it.

Comfort from Pets

I've read many times about how pets keep you calm, how pet owners live longer and generally how beneficial they are to our well-being. Now I've been reflecting on why that might be. My first thought was that it's because they love you. Then I considered our two rather lazy guinea pigs, and wondered if you could really credit them with such an in-depth feeling! I remembered the story of Lester Levenson, and it began to make sense.

Lester was a scientist who became very ill and was expected to die at any time. He realised that he was not going to survive as a result of any external treatment, so turned inside himself to look for answers. The insights he gained now form the basis of The Sedona Method. This is a practical method for dealing with emotions, which you can read more about in the next chapter. The insight I am referring to here is when he realised that his happiness did not depend on others loving him. It depended on whether he was *being loving to others*.

To me, this is the explanation for what we get from pets – we get an opportunity to be loving. It is easier to simply love a pet than a person, as our relationships with them are less clouded by ego.

So if you have pets, make time to spend with them. If not, and you don't want the responsibility of looking after one, find someone who has the kind of pet you like best. (If you don't like any pets, then this isn't for you!) Ask to spend time with your friend's pet. It is a rare person who wouldn't allow you to walk their dog occasionally (which would also get you exercise and time in nature). Even holding someone's guinea pig or rabbit while you visit them for a coffee might do!

Making the Most of Nature

I wonder why it is that so many of us feel better when we're in a natural environment. Perhaps our short years of fast-paced technology haven't managed to overcome centuries of living in tune with the land. Maybe it's because our bodies feel the energy of the sun and the tidal pull of the moon as much as does any plant or ocean.

I've been watching a TV programme made by my local celebrity food writer, Hugh Fearnley-Whittingstall. He works not far from me in the beautiful county of Devon. The programme was promoting the benefits of living in tune with the seasons – in this case Spring. Hugh says this has been one of the joys he's experienced in his last ten years while creating a life where he grows and eats much of his own produce.

Luckily we don't all need to create a smallholding or farm to get the benefits of being in tune with nature. Open spaces of all kinds, including parks in towns and cities, give everyone the opportunity to sit or walk. You can soak up the beauty of a plant, or the clouds in the sky. I now live by the sea, and I see the way it draws people to just stand and watch the waves.

Tending your garden can also be a source of peace and pleasure. If you don't have a garden, there are ways to grow plants in containers in your home or on a balcony. You can even grow tomatoes in a hanging basket!

As well as its beauty, nature has the benefit of bringing you in tune with the seasons, as Hugh said. It gives you a sense of where you fit into that nature. The coast near where I live is known as the Jurassic Coast, as the cliffs are full of fossils of the animals that lived here 65 *million* years ago. That certainly gives me a sense of perspective as to how short a time we humans have been around – and how the world will get on just fine without me one day.

Humour and Pleasure

I already shared with you the saying "What I Focus On Expands", and so it is with our attitude to life. A light-hearted, positive attitude (even amongst the sadness you are feeling) will bring good things into your life. A dear friend once gave me a card with the saying "Angels can fly because they take themselves lightly". What a lovely thought.

You have probably already noticed that although I'm dealing with a 'serious' time in your life, I'm doing so without getting too heavy about it. This is deliberate, and also a true reflection of how I see it. Just because something challenging is happening in your life; that is no reason to stop having fun. Quite the opposite, in fact. You need intense doses of fun and pleasant activities, to offset any negative feelings about your loved one's cancer.

I mentioned before the story of Cathy Goodman, whose healing from breast cancer was featured in *The Secret*. Her healing had three main components: belief that she was healed and seeing that as true; gratitude for that healing; and the power of laughter to heal. Cathy and her husband watched videos of funny movies for months. They avoided any kind of bad news, or anything that could cause her stress. Within three months her cancer was gone, with no other treatment. If laughter has the power to heal physically, it certainly can heal emotionally too. It can keep the positive energy going. That's why we've included a humour section on our forum at www.familiesfacingcancer.org - so you can share what makes you laugh!

Nutrition

At a time like this, you may be likely to let your diet slide a little. After all, I've just told you that you need pleasure in your life. So you do. There's certainly nothing wrong with a few sweets or chocolates, or the odd glass of wine, particularly if it gives you pleasure.

The danger comes if you become too busy to eat properly. If your partner is ill and can't eat regular meals, perhaps you see no point making a proper meal. Maybe it even seems wrong to you to eat a generous helping of anything your loved one can't share. If you get into the 'can't be bothered' cycle, your body will crave fuel, and you may be tempted to grab whatever is easiest. If that happens to be a salad you could do well, but I would hazard a guess that you might choose a chocolate bar instead.

Often we use food as a way of dealing with our emotions – or rather of suppressing them. You can even have specific food cravings linked to the emotions you are feeling, as described in Doreen Virtue's book *Constant Craving*. In other words food can become a way of self-medicating, in just the same way as alcohol or television can. But at this time your body needs good nutrition. It always does, of course, but now the physical and emotional demands on you are greater. Your need for quality fuel to maintain your health is more than it has ever been. If you want to be able to keep at your optimum health, even just so that you can help the cancer host, don't neglect the food you eat. You may also find that your loved one is altering their diet, and joining them in this could be very supportive.

I'm sure you don't need me to tell you that a healthy diet involves more natural food, fruit, vegetables and whole grains - and less processed food, sugar and other empty calories. If you don't have a lot of time to prepare nutritious meals, food is an area where you can get help. If offers of help come in, you can ask for some healthy dinners for your freezer, for those times when you are too tired or emotional to cook.

Extra Expenses

Cancer often brings with it unavoidable extra expenses. Therapies or additional treatments may be available through hospices, or you may have to pay for them.

Trips to hospitals or other centres for treatment can be costly. So can travelling to see your loved one if they live at a distance. You may want to take the person who has cancer away on a holiday at a time when they are well enough to enjoy it, or get away by yourself. Even buying books such as this to support you is an extra expense.

It is likely that there will be more of an effect on you if you have joint finances with the cancer host. Even if you don't, you may worry about the additional expenses your loved one is having to meet. Now, I'm not going to make any assumptions about the state of your finances. I hope that you have plenty of income every month and don't need to worry about a little extra spending, or you have a good cushion of savings to fall back on. What I am saying is that it is important to be aware of your finances - and responsible for them.

Notice where there are extra expenses, and equally if there are any areas where you are spending less – perhaps not going out as much, for instance. If you see that your expenses have gone up by more than you can easily afford, deal with it quickly. Don't wait until you get into financial difficulty to tackle the problem.

This book can't teach you to budget if you're not doing this, but there are lots of other excellent resources that will. You could read *You and Your Money* by Alvin Hall, or use some kind of budgeting software such as *Quicken*.

Finally, don't be too proud to accept offers of help that

benefit you financially. If there is someone who is longing to help, can't be there in person but has plenty of spare money, maybe they would love to pay for a holiday for the cancer host. They would be contributing the resource they have available. Why not let them?

Avoiding Financial Difficulty

This follows on from the issue of extra expenses. Usually it will occur when the cancer host is unable to continue to work – or if you have to give up work to care for them.

Once upon a time, not all that long ago, most people worked in secure jobs for many years. They had full sickness cover, and their wages would continue to be paid if they became ill. For many that situation no longer exists. When my mother became ill, her employment contract had just been renewed for a year. Her pay would have lasted only as long as that contract.

Sick pay generally goes down over time, rather than staying at the same level as previous earnings. Your loved one may also lose any part of their pay that was based on commission, performance or overtime. If the cancer host contributed a major part of their household income, and this is affected, problems could arise.

The most important thing, of course, is to face up to facts as soon as they become clear. Plan ahead of time what you (or they, if you are not part of their household) can do to deal with the problem. It seems ironic that just as expenses are probably rising, their ability to cover those expenses is threatened.

It is possible that the person with cancer has some kind of insurance that covers this situation. They can dig it out and check the terms and conditions. Some policies cover illness, and others will pay out early if the person is not expected to live. You have to be practical if your finances are threatened, even if you don't like facing up to unpleasant facts.

Some help may be available from outside agencies. You could have a list of these in your Plan. Contact them to see if help is available in your situation. The person with cancer may be able to claim some welfare benefits to help out. This is often a long process, so don't leave it until a financial crisis is upon you.

Some also choose to tap into equity they have built up in their home to tide them over this time. This could be done: through an equity release scheme; by moving to a cheaper property; or by using a 'Sell and Rent Back' company.

Be sure to check out the companies you deal with. Compare the end results carefully, and take financial advice if you need it in order to understand the full implications.

Using Your Support System

Although I have talked about your support system in earlier chapters, this has mostly been in terms of emotional support. But don't underestimate how much practical help you need, or how much is available. Many people you know will want to be able to help. Giving them something practical they can do for you or the cancer host will really help them to feel better. There is no greater satisfaction than selfless giving, so who are you to deny them this pleasure?

There are many different areas in which you can receive practical help. These include :

- Nursing help, which may be provided through cancer charities, or privately.

- Someone to sit with the cancer host and give a carer a break or time to sleep.

- Cooking meals.

- Paying for a holiday or a therapy treatment.

- Handling enquiries from the rest of the family (see the next section).

- Doing some washing or cleaning.

- Transport to or from hospital or other appointments.

- Taking on responsibility for personal or business paperwork.

- Doing research and finding information.

- Searching out funny videos or stories.

Many more ideas can be found in the book *What Can I Do To Help? : 75 Practical Ideas For Family And Friends From Cancer's Frontline*, by Deborah Hutton.

The key is to be prepared when people offer their assistance. If you think in advance "What could we use some help with?" then you will have a list available. You will be able to include this in your Cancer Success Plan. This will also prepare you mentally for expecting help – which we often find difficult. When someone says to you "Can I do anything to help", your mouth may well automatically say "No, no, we're doing fine" before your brain has time to step in. So rehearse as you create your list. You could reply "Well, thanks for offering. You know, we could use a little help with . . .". It is important to accept some help when it is offered, or at least set that up for the future. The chances are that if you turn down an offer of help, that person won't offer again. However, if you say to them "We're okay at the moment, but can I call you if we need help in the future?" then you have left that door open. You could even talk about the type of help they would be able to give in the future.

Also bear in mind that help for you is just as valid as that for the cancer host. You are important too. You will also be better able to support your loved one if pressure is taken off you.

Dealing with the Rest of the World

Once people around you know there has been a diagnosis of cancer, there will be an insatiable appetite for information, particularly amongst those who know the cancer host. If you live with the person who has cancer, you may find yourself endlessly answering the telephone and relating the same details to one relative after another. If you live at a distance, you may be one of the people phoning – and possibly feeling guilty about doing so. It's important to handle this communication issue, as it can drive the sanest person to distraction.

The most important factor is to set down some boundaries about the best ways to communicate. Is email easier, because you can choose when to reply? Do you, or the cancer host, like to chat on the phone - but only at certain times? Would you prefer to update one person, and have them pass the information around the family for you?

If you are the one desperately wanting an update, but find it hard to get information, ask the cancer host or others in the family what would work best for them.

One way that a family can come together for mutual support at a time like this is to build a private website. This way people with fresh information can update it so that everyone can read it. If you have a question, you can ask it there, and get an answer from anyone who knows what you are seeking. You can share positive stories, family news, happy memories, and even photos. If you have a family member in their teens or twenties, they will probably know how to create this much better than I do – and feel good about being involved. If not, you can learn to set up a website through Wordpress, or use the system provided at www.caringbridge.org.

Focus on the Future

There is a wonderful saying "Plan as if you will live forever – live as if you will die tomorrow." What that means is that you expect the best from tomorrow and then get the most you can out of today in case that doesn't happen.

My husband's grandfather lived into his nineties, yet the year before he died he was still looking forward. "I think I ought to have a new suit this year", he said, and "The fruit trees will need pruning in the spring."

This confidence in there being a tomorrow was inspiring, and I'm sure it contributed to his long life. In contrast we have other relatives who refuse to plan a holiday for next year in case they are not around then. I know which attitude would serve me best, and I make an effort to emulate Pap, as we knew him.

So whilst you are dealing with the practical problems and issues that arise on this journey, keep the destination you want firmly in your mind. You can even spend time visualising how you would like everything to turn out. Bear in mind that this situation, and the journey you are on, is temporary. It will probably be a small portion of your whole life, but it can be a significant one if you are brave enough to take the Inner Journey.

ACTION STEP

Set aside a time, and if possible a space, for yourself some time in the next week. Write it in your calendar or diary as an appointment with yourself. If you break this appointment, for whatever reason, then make the appointment again for a time within three days.

If you break the appointment a second time, then give a sum of money (say the amount that it would cost you for an expensive meal out) or some time to charity – but it must be a charity you dislike, so that you have a real incentive to keep your appointment.

6

THE INNER JOURNEY – EMOTIONS AND SPIRIT

The part of the journey you *have* to make was covered in the last chapter – all the practical issues you may have to deal with.

In this chapter, we will delve a little deeper. We'll look at the emotions that can come up for you, and how best to deal with them. Many people get through their experience by suppressing their emotions and ignoring that part of their journey. On the surface this may seem to be a successful approach. Usually, though, these emotions turn up again at a later time, causing more damage. The way to avoid this is to have the courage to take this inner journey now. Are you ready?

First we will look at some of the reasons that strong emotions are arising at this time. Then we'll find some of the ways and means you can use to deal successfully with how you feel.

Seeing Changes in Your Loved One

One cause that is likely to create strong emotions for you is the changes that you may see in the cancer host. This person you love is going through a challenging time, and it is likely to have an impact on the way they look and behave.

To see a parent ageing before your eyes can be an uncomfortable experience. A beloved partner who no longer wants to be held or caressed because touch is uncomfortable can make you feel like they have rejected your love. If a favourite uncle turns from cheerfulness to complaining, it can seem as though you have lost the real person already. Don't deny the feelings that come up for you. Notice how you feel, and admit when you find it hard. Ways for dealing with the feelings you find are given later in this chapter.

Try as well to remember that the real person is still there inside what you see. When we look at someone we don't only see what's on the surface. It has been said that the eyes are the windows of the soul – so you see much of the real person in their eyes. So remember to look for the real person underneath the changes. Perhaps then you will find your emotions easier to deal with.

Saying the Wrong Thing

Shock can make people say the most appalling things. In the UK we have an expression 'open mouth and insert foot' – very strange I know. I'm not sure why we refer to saying something insensitive as 'putting our foot in it' (although it may have a farming connection), but we do. Sometimes it doesn't even have to be caused by shock, just by not thinking before speaking.

You will probably find that many people say 'the wrong thing' to you. I could quite possibly be one of them. You could get horribly offended about that. You could even tell yourself for years about how thoughtless they have been. If this has already happened to you, then pause for a moment. Can you remember a time when you said something you regretted? It could have been in an interview, or the heat of an argument. You probably knew it was the wrong thing to say almost at once. Did you apologise and fix the issue then, or let it fester until later?

None of us is immune from saying something that could cause offence, so don't punish someone who makes that mistake. Tell yourself "Oh, they didn't mean it like that." Then let it go and move on. If it's a big issue, and you can't do that yet, then talk to them. The person may not even realise they offended you, and may quickly be able to make amends. Just be aware of the advice often given to couples. Don't attack the person for their mistake, this will only put them on the defensive. Instead, talk in terms of how their comments made you feel. Don't be attached to how they respond, just know that you've let it out and let it go.

Another problem that can occur is if you become scared of saying the wrong thing to your loved one. You may dumb down your conversations with them for fear of offending with your words. Doing this, though, is far worse than making a blunder. What your loved one needs more than ever is to be able to communicate with you. They can't do this if you are watching your words so much that you don't say what you really feel.

So please don't hold on to things that others say to you, especially when emotions are running high. This will free you to speak fearlessly as well. If you *have* said something you regret, let the person know. Forgive yourself first, and then tell them what you wish you had said or done.

Resentment of Attention Focused Elsewhere

As I mentioned in Chapter 3, you may find many feelings come up for you that relate to a desire for attention. You are not the only person to feel that way. You don't need to feel guilty about it, but it is as well to notice these emotions. You could write about why you feel so strongly. Does the situation remind you of a time in the past when you felt shut out? Or have you always had lots of attention and resent its removal all the more?

I had a time at school when only two girls in the class would speak to me. They didn't sit near me in class, so I felt really isolated. This can make me rather sensitive to being ignored, because it tends to hit a nerve. I am now more aware of the problem, and have a coping strategy. I have friends who do care about what I have to say, with whom I can get in touch if I need someone to listen to me.

Don't deny the way you feel, but stay aware when resentment creeps in. Head it off by making sure you take care of yourself. When you give yourself enough attention, you will be less dependent on finding it from outside sources.

Bringing up Buried Feelings

My experience of being ignored in school also shows how things that have happened in the past can come back to haunt us today. If we were all completely enlightened we would live in the moment, and past hurts and fears would have no influence on us. But then, of course, there would have been little point in writing this book for you. In reality, things that happened yesterday or many years ago still affect us all the time – often without our even being conscious of the fact.

Some of the hardest emotions you might have to face would be if you haven't fully dealt with feelings about losing someone close to you in the past. These feelings could be especially strong if that person died of cancer.

Perhaps you have had cancer yourself in the past, and your fears come rushing back. This was the case for my mother-in-law when my husband's aunt, Trudi, became ill. She feared once again for her own health at the same time as worrying about Trudi. Any feelings you suppressed at the time are likely to resurface now. Any emotional issues that haven't been dealt with in your relationship with the cancer host may also be made worse at this time.

The first thing to recognise is that emotions are not *bad* things. They're not particularly *good* things either. What they are is a message. Unless they are happy emotions, they are a message that something needs to be dealt with - like a signpost on your journey. So the resurfacing of old emotions is an opportunity.

I once read in an article featured in the *Cygnus Review* (a magazine and book catalogue) that unless you expose mud to the sunlight it can never dry out. So all those old muddy emotions need to come to the surface. Your inner journey will provide the sunlight that dries up the mud. Then you will no longer be bogged down in those particular feelings.

Dealing with Anger

Anger is one of the most damaging of all emotions. We hear and read a lot about road rage, but anger can occur in many other situations. Feeling fury can be terrifying. You are convinced that the anger will consume you, and there will be nothing else left. When you are tired, stressed and worried, anger often arises more easily.

A long wait to pay at the shop can send you spiralling into a fury far beyond what is reasonable. I'm sure you've seen someone yelling at an assistant over some seemingly insignificant problem. Their anger is probably not much to do with the current issue; it's more likely related to what kind of day they've had, or what kind of person they are.

Feeling anger is one level of problem, but the more important issue is what we do with it. Those shop assistants do not deserve the fury that's being aimed at them, but they are on the receiving end of it. If you vent your anger at someone, you can't take back the things you said – and that is dangerous. When you are angry, you can damage your relationships with those around you.

All these things mean that we are scared of feeling anger. We're not good at dealing with it, as we have not been taught how to. Instead we tend to suppress those angry feelings, because this seems safer than allowing ourselves to feel that way. In fact what you are doing by suppressing anger is choosing to hang on to it. You may have heard the expression "What you resist, persists", and so it is with those feelings of fury.

Of course I'm not recommending that you let it out and shout at people in shops, but there are many safer ways of expressing feelings – or even just dropping them, as you will see below in **Ways and Means**.

Confronting Your Own Mortality

Are you at peace with the idea of your own death? Often those who are really at the point of death do feel great peace. They stop fighting, and their fear is gone. Thinking of your own death from a distance can be much harder. We often have a fierce attachment to our lives here. We've got things to do, people to look after, places to visit and money to make. Life seems much too short to fit it all in.

When someone close to you faces such a major illness, it can cause you to dwell on the possibility of death. This may not be something you are used to doing. Many people find death almost impossible to think about, even to the extent where they are unable to make a will. That would mean admitting death is sure to happen one day! You may feel your life is pointless if one day you will cease to exist.

You may fear that at death you will be 'judged' for every minor error or major sin you committed during your life. My belief is that whatever higher power is out there (or within you) has already judged you to be perfect, and regards your faults as minor interruptions in the true you. If you have a strong sense of self or a spiritual belief, this may allow you to feel confident that the essence of yourself continues after death. This could be as spirit, through your life achievements, or living on in the hearts of others. This can be a comfort when you feel a fear of your own death arising.

In the end, there is nothing to be gained from dwelling on when or if you are going to die. It is inevitable. If you want to focus on still being here, consider this quote from the book *Illusions* by Richard Bach: "Here is a test to find whether your mission on earth is finished: if you're alive, it isn't."

So don't focus on your eventual death. It is irrelevant now. You get to choose the mission you are on, though it would be as well to include learning and laughter at its centre. As Michel de Montaigne said "The value of life lies not in the length of days, but in the use we make of them."

Stop Pretending You're OK

You can't deal with emotions by pretending they don't exist. I know you want to be positive, to look forward and manifest the best possible result for yourself and your loved one. And you will. But plastering a happy face on top of a sea of negativity, fear and doubt is not going to do the trick. When someone asks you "How are you?" how do you react? "Oh, I'm fine thanks"? Sometimes I've phoned my sister and asked this question, but the tone of her reply sounded exactly the opposite of what she said.

In order to work, positive thinking has to be genuine. It's like doing that old self-development favourite – affirmations. You can stand in front of the mirror saying "I am slim" all you like - but that affirmation will never work if at the same time your mind is keeping up a dialogue about how you're a liar. On the other hand, if you have let go of negative emotions about your weight; if you truly see your slender self out there in the future, that affirmation will bring it to you faster.

When someone asks how you are, or you're writing in your private journal, be true to how you feel. Don't hold on to those feelings, but acknowledge them. You might want to say something like, "Well, I'm having a tough time at the moment with Tim being ill, but we're pulling together as a family".

If you really are at your wits' end then say so – you may get some help as a result. After all, why would anyone step in to assist if you're giving the impression that you can handle everything yourself?

Who is Your Emotional Sounding Board?

One outside resource that can help you in dealing with your feelings is what I call an emotional sounding board. This is a person, or several people, who will listen to how you feel. They could be a friend, family member or colleague, someone on a help line or at a support centre, your spiritual adviser, a professional counsellor or life coach.

To be a successful sounding board, they should satisfy these conditions:

- They see you and the person who has cancer as capable, not as victims.
- They can take the tough stuff, and won't crumble if you're talking about challenging issues.
- They aren't personally affected by your loved one's cancer.

- They are able to let you express how you feel without jumping in with unwanted 'fixes'.

Having an emotional sounding board will allow you to be more in control as to how and when you express your emotions. You could arrange regular meetings or phone calls, or contact your sounding board when you need them. However, this isn't an excuse to dwell on emotions, or indulge in endless sessions moaning about your lot! Make sure the focus is on getting the emotions out and gone.

Your Feelings Affect Others

Do you remember my relatives from Chapter 5? The ones who won't book a holiday for next year in case they're not around any more. Well I have to confess, we don't visit them often. I remember one time sitting in their kitchen, chatting. Everything we mentioned, they responded to with a tale of doom and gloom. When we left, I looked at my husband with utter relief. We felt as though we had spent the afternoon being pressed under a dark blanket of misery. That's why we only visit occasionally, and then keep the topic of conversation as light as we can.

Just as those people affect how I feel, so *your* emotions will affect those around you. Now, this doesn't mean that you're totally responsible for how they feel. I am perfectly able to shrug off the dark blanket and choose not to let it continue to affect me. Your effect is still something you can be aware of, though.

When you live with someone, it is especially difficult to be unaffected by their emotions. Children in particular are like sponges, absorbing the energy of those around them.

All your close friends and family are on their own journey, including the cancer host. They have their own torrent of emotions - and are dealing with them in their own way, doing the best they can. You owe it to everyone to deal with your emotions.

Don't be afraid of sharing how you feel, just be an example. Do what you need to do to work with those feelings, process them and let them go. You can become an oasis of peace, calm and strength, with a positive effect on those around you.

Acceptance or Resistance

A diagnosis of cancer feels like bad news, doesn't it? How do people react when they hear bad news? "No way", "You're joking", "I can't believe it" are the kind of thing you might hear, or say. What they have in common is resistance. We don't want the news to be true, so we try to push it away with our words and thoughts. Perhaps if we pretend hard enough, hum loudly or look the other way it will stop being true. Do you think it will? Of course not.

Resisting the truth takes a lot of energy, though. You have to concentrate fiercely on something else in order to block out what's happening. You might be tempted to self-medicate using TV, alcohol, drugs or food to block out your unwelcome thoughts. None of these are healthy pursuits if you use them to excess.

Even though you have spent all that energy, you will not reduce your belief in the bad news one bit. In fact by resisting, you have made it seem all the more real. The 'War on Cancer', which was declared by President Nixon in 1971, has done exactly this. So has the

'War on Terror' and the 'War on Drugs'. The cynic in me suspects that politicians create these great resistances just as, in days of old, (and indeed more recently) they would invade their neighbours to divert the attention of the people from problems at home.

Our worst fear is that if we accept something as true (like the cancer), that we are somehow giving in. We fear that we will become passive - but this need not be the case. By accepting the current situation, what you do is free up all that energy you were using to resist. Then you can put it into a more positive effort. In fact what we are really resisting is not the situation, anyway, but our *unwelcome feelings* about the situation.

The ways and means described below will help you dissolve that resistance. Also, both The Sedona Method and Byron Katie's The Works (described in her book *Loving What Is*) explore resistance in some detail, and give methods for dealing with it.

The 'Gift' of Cancer

Whilst I was looking up one of the quotes I used earlier, I came across another one. Again it's from *Illusions* by Richard Bach, and it says, "There is no such thing as a problem without a gift for you in its hands." Now, I know you have not sought the problem of your loved one's cancer. You would possibly even prefer to have cancer yourself than to watch them suffer. But, coming unrequested as it has, the problem has brought with it an opportunity.

I once had a neighbour, José, who was diagnosed with a brain tumour. A chronic workaholic, he had been putting off all his enjoyment whilst he built his accountancy business. What José said to me was, "Although I don't want to die, I'm glad I got cancer, because it made me realise what is important in my life." José is not alone in using his cancer to realise where the deeper meaning of his life lay. Many people take this journey.

The good news for you is that you don't have cancer, but you still have the same opportunity to learn. You can look at your relationships, how you balance the commitments in your life, and what you are doing to make yourself happy. In fact I think this is so fundamental that some day I'm going to write a book called *How To Learn Life's Lessons – Without Waiting Until You Get Ill!* This is why the Inner Journey is so worthwhile. By taking it you can ensure that you have accepted the 'gift' of this problem. Then the hard times will not have been in vain.

Get to Know Your Loved One More Deeply

While the situation you are in can be used as a lens to look clearly at the whole of your life, there is one area in particular in which it can really make a difference. That is in your relationship with the person who has cancer. If you already have a good relationship, you will be amazed at how much deeper it can become. If you don't, you now have an opportunity to address the problems.

Whilst writing this book, I have told lots of new people about my mother dying. Often they ask "Were you close?" - as if that meant it hurt more, or less, to lose her. The truth is that we weren't – before the cancer. One of my aunts once told me that she thought I was very like Mum in her younger days. Perhaps that is why her disapproval of some of my life decisions was so strong, and why I never felt quite good enough for her.

My mother's illness, for us, was an opening. Her attitude to me seemed to change, and certainly my attitude to her did. It was no longer important to defend my decisions or actions, only to build some kind of connection before it was too late. Of course, I now realise that it is never too late. If you are prepared to really hear your loved one, you will continue to learn about them even if they have died, as you remember old conversations.

If you let go of being attached to your end of the relationship; if you can forget about what you are getting out of it and just give, then you will have the space to feel your connection with your loved one either in person or in spirit.

Ways and Means

So far we've noted that you are dealing with some strong emotions. They may come up because of changes you see in your loved one, because someone says the wrong thing, because you resent attention being taken away from you, from the resurfacing of feelings you have buried, from confronting your own mortality or because you are resisting the situation.

I have suggested that you can use this difficult situation as a tool for your own personal growth and as a way to get to know and love the cancer host more deeply. Now it's time to look further at ways you can deal with your emotions, and achieve that growth.

The first step to being able to deal with emotions is to stop assigning labels to them. I already said that feelings are neither 'good' nor 'bad'. Having those feelings also doesn't make you a 'good person' or a 'bad person'. There are no judgements for feelings. They are simply based on thoughts you are having for a brief moment. You can choose to keep those thoughts and continue the feelings, or you can find ways to let those thoughts and feelings pass through you.

You may want to use some or all of the following methods. There is no right or wrong way. Just start with the one you feel most drawn to, and carry on from there. You will find all of these covered in the rest of this chapter:

- Keeping a journal
- Meditation
- Creativity
- Release through humour
- Sedona Method
- Therapies
- Healing emotions in relationships
- Physical exercise
- Counselling
- Life coaching
- Prayer
- Open your heart

Keeping a journal

On the surface, journalling is a very simple process. You write about the things that happen to you, and how you feel about them. The process of writing is very interesting, though, because you can use it to tap into your subconscious feelings. (You need to choose not to let your brain edit what you write.) Journalling helps you to let go of emotions because it is a safe way of expressing feelings without having to act on them. You may well find that simply writing about how you feel will reduce the strength of those feelings. If writing them down makes you cry, this is probably helpful, as tears are a wonderful release.

The simplest version of this kind of journalling would be to create a Hard Times Notebook, as recommended by Barbara Sher in her book *Wishcraft*. This will give you somewhere to complain, and to dump all your unwanted feelings. If you want a deeper level of journalling, and to really explore your inner landscape, you can do that as well. You can find your own approach, or if you're not sure where to start you could read *Journalution* by Sandy Grason. This will give you an in depth guide to how journalling can support your inner journey.

Meditation

Teachers frequently recommend meditation, whatever situation you have in your life. Its benefits are many and varied. You can improve your health through meditation, potentially lowering your blood pressure for instance. People who meditate regularly tend to be calmer and more peaceful to be around. The effects spread beyond the person who is actually meditating. In fact a study in Washington DC showed that a group of 4,000 people in the city meditating on a daily basis for 8 weeks resulted in the rate of violent crime falling by over 20% (and this doesn't mean that the people who were meditating committed fewer crimes!). The purpose of meditating is to clear out the mental chatter that goes on in our brains when we're not watching – or at least to notice it and stop identifying with it.

How would you start to meditate if you're not doing it already? You may be utterly bewildered by the many different methods and systems that people use to meditate. Every single one is valid, so it's just a matter of finding one that makes sense to you. Some methods recommend focusing on breathing, or simply noticing your thoughts. Some involve repeating a word or sound (Transcendental Meditation for instance), or perhaps humming. Others say that meditation can be 'intentional', where you set a purpose or goal for your meditation. You could also use visualisation techniques.

Meditation can also take place during daily activities that don't involve a lot of thinking. Even doing the dishes can be a meditative process if you quieten your mind. One way of doing this is to concentrate fully on the task. When stray thoughts about the past or future crop up, watch them and let them go, then return to the task at hand. This is a very peaceful way to get through your chores.

If you want help in beginning to meditate, you could join a local group, or buy one of the many meditation tools that are on the market. My sister recommends the book *Moon Over Water* by Jessica Williams Macbeth as an excellent place to start.

Creativity

Just as writing can help you tap into your subconscious, so can other forms of creativity. Arthur Koestler said, "Creative activity could be described as a type of learning process where teacher and pupil are located in the same individual." At its extreme this is art therapy, but you might prefer just to think of it as a creative outlet.

Even people who think they are not artistic at all have produced some moving works of art. (Especially when they stopped judging themselves and what they created.) That said, you don't have to share with anyone if you don't want to. All you need to do is find your kind of creativity. The simplest is probably a pencil and paper, but felt pens, paints, clay, fabric or card and glue can all be used. Colour does add a fun element. Blythe House Hospice have a lovely piece of artwork on their walls which is simply hand prints of all those in the group at the time - which each then decorated with painted rings, fingernails etc. as they chose.

Keep in mind that the purpose of your creation is to express how you feel. You could even have a picture that you add to in many sessions as your journey unfolds. That could be an interesting project, seeing how your art grows along your journey.

Release through humour

Humour is a wonderful way to defuse tension, and let go of emotions. Many people who have cancer develop a black sense of humour, and this allows them to deal with really tough times and emotions.

My friend Annette Shaw once supported her neighbour through cancer treatment. She described her experiences, writing in *The Times*. Trying to encourage her friend, Annette thought of telling her about the visualisation techniques where you see your white blood cells as soldiers attacking the cancer 'invaders'. "Think of it as Custer's Last Stand", she concluded triumphantly. "Nette", said her friend, "he lost!" The look of horror on Annette's face provoked gales of laughter from her friend. The ice was broken, and humour kept them both going through many dark hours.

You too can find things to laugh about – even in the face of hardship. There is definitely a funny side to the indignities of cancer. Obviously I'm not inviting you to laugh at your loved one, but if they can find humour then respond. They may be longing for someone to be light-hearted around them. It's hard to hold on to anger, fear and even despair if you are laughing.

Sedona Method

The Sedona Method is absolutely one of the best methods of dealing directly with your own emotions that I have ever come across. You don't need to believe anything in particular. You don't have to have a therapist to help you. You can do it with your eyes open, your clothes on, and even in a crowded room. It is so easy that everyone can learn it, but you could practise it for a lifetime.

Lester Levenson developed this simple and easy method for his own use. It is now taught by Hale Dwoskin (who you may have seen in the film *The Secret*), and Sedona Training Associates. The Sedona Method is based on the principle that as children we naturally let go of emotions and let them pass through us. I was once told that the definition of emotion was energy in motion. But we have learned to hold on to our feelings, stop the movement, and that is what keeps us stuck. The Sedona Method is a series of questions that helps you remember how to let go of emotions in order to uncover the underlying peace you have at your core. You can find out more about the Sedona Method at www.sedona.com.

Therapies

I already described in the last chapter how complementary therapies can help with handling stress and maintaining energy levels. All the therapies mentioned there, and many more, can also be of benefit in your emotional journey.

My sister is a massage therapist and tells me that in her treatments it is not uncommon for clients to become emotional, even to cry. This allows them to release feelings they have been holding on to.

Another therapy you might like to consider, in addition to those listed in Chapter 5, is the Emotional Freedom Technique. This technique involves using acupressure points (which you tap lightly with your fingers) in order to release deep emotional problems. It is something you can explore on your own, or with a practitioner. For more information about this and other therapies than I have room for here, you can visit our website at www.familiesfacingcancer.org.

Healing emotions in relationships

It may be a bit less clear how relationships are a way of releasing emotions, so let me explain what I mean.

When you are feeling any emotion, you are thinking mainly of yourself. For instance, you can't be shy while fully focusing on someone else. If you choose to take the focus off yourself, though, and direct it to your relationship with someone else, the strength of the emotion can be reduced.

Your emotions do matter, but wallowing in them doesn't help. Getting to know the people around you better, caring about them and listening to how they feel are all ways to focus attention outside yourself. In doing so, you will feel less need to hold on to your feelings, and may find you let go of them naturally.

Physical exercise

One of the places we hold emotions is in our bodies. We hunch our shoulders when we are nervous, ball up our fists when we are angry and slump in our chairs in despair. Your emotions are completely connected to your body. It's why you get told to stand tall to overcome a lack of confidence. Changing your posture can change the way you feel. So another way to help you with your emotions is to use physical exercise.

The type of exercise you choose may depend on what your main emotions are. If you feel angry, energetic sports can be a release. If your main emotion is sadness, perhaps a long walk or some yoga would seem more suitable. The reverse could also be true – kickboxing could demolish sadness and yoga dissolve your fury. And perhaps going dancing would be an even better antidote for all woes.

Counselling

Traditionally problems relating mainly to emotions have been dealt with by counselling. It is well known as a support for people who have depression, for couples with relationship issues, and in the case of bereavement.

A counsellor can discuss your situation with you, encourage you to talk about how you feel, or simply sit with you in whatever emotion you are experiencing.

If you find that the other methods described here are not enough to help you handle your emotions, you might want to visit a counsellor. This may be especially the case if your emotions are making it difficult for you to get through your everyday life for a long time. It is quite normal to find it hard to deal with your work for a time when you have had an emotional upset. If you are unable to adjust after weeks or even months, this is a time to seek help. This is even more true if you feel you may be slipping into depression. You could find a counsellor through your doctor, or hire one privately.

Life coaching

Life coaches take a slightly different approach from counsellors. They help you to look at your whole life rather than just the issue you are dealing with. They are likely to encourage you to look at the life you would like to move towards more than at the problems you have had in the past – though they will look with you at how those problems still affect you today. Life coaching is a very positive approach, both to dealing with the emotions you have now and to finding ways to improve all areas of your life in the future. A trained coach will ask questions that allow you to discover the wisdom you already have about what is right for you.

With coaching, you are in the driving seat, and your coach is like the satnav, or route map, that helps you to take the turns to get to your chosen destination. Correcting when you take a wrong turn is part of the process. At Families Facing Cancer, we offer a support service that uses coaching skills to guide you through your journey. You can find out more about the programmes on offer at www.familiesfacingcancer.org.

Prayer

Times of deep emotion and challenge can rock your faith. How can a loving God visit such pain on someone you love? On the other hand these situations can strengthen your faith. They could even create the drive for you to return to a faith you have let slide of late. If you are open to faith and prayer, they can be a source of great strength for you. They can help you in handling your emotions, and give a stability that underpins your whole life.

You might also want to know that some studies have shown improved recovery rates in people who were prayed for. It didn't matter whether the patients in the study knew they were being prayed for, or the belief system of those doing the praying (so long as they believed they could make a difference). The one thing that most improved the outcome was that those praying should ask not for the person's recovery, but for their best possible outcome, whatever that might be.

If you want to pray for your loved one as well as for your own strength, simply make sure you are not relying on a particular outcome. This has been described as 'Let go and let God'. If you want to pray, but are unsure what to say, you could always use the *Serenity Prayer* written by Reinhold Niebuhr:

"God grant me

the serenity to accept the things I cannot change,

the courage to change the things I can,

and wisdom to know the difference."

Open your heart

Some people react to heartache by closing themselves off. They feel that if they refuse to let themselves love, they won't be able to be hurt, but how wrong they are. What they are losing – and the hurt they are causing themselves – is far worse than even the pain of losing someone you love. I hope you won't be tempted to be one of them.

Always remember that there can be no rainbow without rain clouds. If you are able to keep your heart open whatever the challenges, I am sure you will find your own rainbow there.

ACTION STEP

Create a journal, Hard Times Notebook or a prayer book, and begin writing in it on a daily basis, or whenever you feel the need. Then add in any other methods of dealing with emotions you feel will be of benefit to you.

7

WHEN THE GOING GETS TOUGH

I hope your journey goes well. Everything you have learned in the previous chapters, combined with your own inner wisdom, will go a long way towards making this happen. But what happens if everything doesn't go according to plan? What if you find the stress becoming too much for you? What if outside forces are taking your life into a more challenging landscape?

Viktor Frankl said "When we can no longer change a situation, we are challenged to change ourselves." As he gained his insights in the concentration camps of wartime Germany, I think he has experienced situations far more challenging than I ever have.

So how do you face up to hard truths and change yourself when you can no longer change the situation?

Firstly you need to do what you can to keep going regardless of the strain. Secondly you need to allow yourself time to make that inner transformation. The rest of this chapter will cover these aspects.

Use Your Preparation

When the going gets tough, when you feel really up against it, when you sink into the depths of despair – these are the times to fall back on the preparations you made before.

By now you will have practised asking for help, or at least accepting the offers that were made. You will have a variety of helpers whom you can call on in the future. Well, now that future is here! Don't wait until you are at your wits' end before you call in the reserves. Do it as soon as you begin to struggle. It is easier to ask someone to visit your loved one for a few hours a week than to ask them to take over from a full-time carer who has had a breakdown.

Turn back to the resources section of your Cancer Success Plan. Remind yourself of what is on hand in the various areas of support. Take a deep breath, and ask for help. If you haven't prepared enough and don't know where to turn, don't give up. Write down what help you could use. Then see where inspiration takes you, or who shows up in your life.

Turn to Hobbies and Outside Interests

I already touched on hobbies and outside interests in Chapter 5. Remember the pigeon fancier whose wife had Alzheimer's disease? His birds helped keep him sane, and your hobbies can do the same for you. It may be tempting to give up all your other pastimes in order to devote all your time and energy to the person who is ill. This may be particularly true if they are declining, and you wonder if they are going to recover.

Your hobbies are part of you, though. They feed your soul, and help you to keep going. If you are the main carer, I would rather you asked for help to look after the cancer host and kept up your other interests, than that you abandoned everything through some misplaced sense of duty or even guilt.

You see, I know a secret. I know you are not selfish. There is a fabulous book called *The Selfish Pig's Guide To Caring*, by Hugh Marriott. The reason this book can get away with such a clever, funny and challenging title is that it is a joke. Carers are *not* selfish – quite the opposite. They do things that are beyond what anybody would or could expect. They go the extra mile and put their loved ones first, often at the expense of themselves. It has been estimated that full time carers provide care which would otherwise cost the UK government £87 billion per year (I can't even contemplate what it must come to worldwide). There are many health issues other than cancer that result in full time care being needed - but if you are playing even a small part in saving those billions, then surely you are entitled to a few hours off every now and then.

Another aspect of outside interests that you may not have faced up to is the benefits they can bring if your loved one dies. They can provide a real sense of stability. You mix with people who know you as John the model maker or Mary the expert potter, not as someone who is almost a part of the cancer host. That can continue, whatever the outcome of your journey.

If the Cancer Returns

Being given a second diagnosis of cancer is very different from the first time. The first time a person gets cancer, they often have a lot of fight in them. That may also be true for a repeat diagnosis, but often the person feels different – and so may you.

The first time cancer is diagnosed anything is possible, even if the diagnosis is given at a late stage. If your loved one has been given a second cancer diagnosis then that means they recovered the first time around. It may be that they can recover again; but it could be harder for them both physically and emotionally. Physically they may be exhausted from their earlier treatments, with their immune system at a low. Emotionally they may also be weary, tired of fighting. Your loved one may dread beginning again on the round of treatment they have endured in the past. My mother-in-law has said she's not sure she could face up to going through the chemotherapy again, especially as she knows all too well what to expect. Of course no one can say now how she would really feel if that day came.

It can be much harder for the cancer host (and you) to find hope the second time around in the face of proof that their earlier recovery did not last. The further diagnosis shows that not all cancer cells had been destroyed, or that the body wasn't able to prevent further cancer developing. You may both feel that the outlook is different this time, but don't assume that all is lost. The cancer host may be able to try a different approach and get better results.

It is little wonder that the cancer host may feel gloomy in this situation, and this can be challenging for you. You might feel they should show the same fight and resolve they did before – after all if they beat the disease once then they can again. But don't blame them if they can't feel that way. It may seem to the cancer host that their earlier treatments only bought them time, not a cure. They could be unsure whether it is worth suffering those treatments again, if the cancer is going to get them sooner or later anyway.

Your loved one has the right to have those thoughts, weigh up those options and make that decision. If they are tired of fighting; if they are ready to let go; if they want to simply die with dignity, then that is their decision – however hard you may find it.

If someone does feel like that, they may find it hard to tell you so. They may believe they are letting you, or the medical team down. My mother felt a little like this after my father paid for them to attend the Bristol Cancer Centre (now Penny Brohn Cancer Care). She worried that he had spent a lot of money for them to go to the Centre, and thought she was letting him down somehow by not recovering.

In this type of situation, it will help if you have already built up a relationship where your loved one can say absolutely anything. The greatest gift you can give someone who feels this way is to hear what they say, and be open and honest with them in return. If they are able to make this a conscious choice, they will feel they have some control. With that power of choice, even their death can be improved. I will cover this more deeply later on in this chapter, under **Being Told it's 'Terminal'**.

Be Prepared for Physical Deterioration

It is very hard to watch someone decline physically. Even though you keep the real them firmly fixed in your mind's eye, there can be no denying what you see. This can be especially shocking if you are not able to see your loved one regularly. The difference in their condition may be more marked from one visit to the next.

This was the case for me with my mother. When she was diagnosed she looked just as she had always done, but a few months later her appearance had altered radically. First her face changed from the effects of her medicines. Later on she seemed to shrink in on herself, as is often the case with very elderly people, though Mum was only 54 years old. I don't believe these changes are just down to physical reasons. It seems to me that a lot of it is due to the lessening of what I would describe as their presence. This relates to something I already described - how you can see the person inside, not just their physical features.

When my first mother-in-law died, it was very sudden. She was a small lady, but somehow I never really noticed that, as she was always so full of life. It was shocking to me how small a bundle she made as they carried her from the house after she died, no longer animated by her personality.

If your loved one is fading, comfort yourself that it is because they are less attached to their body. This will make things easier for them, and you.

Consider Whether You can Manage at Home

I am going to write this section as if you are living with the cancer host. If you are not, but know someone who is, then all these points may apply to them. If they haven't read this book for themselves, you may want to talk to them about these issues.

If the person who has cancer is becoming unable to care for themselves, this has huge implications for those who live with them. This could be their spouse, their child or their parent. Whatever the relationship, caring for someone round the clock is not something to take on lightly. Allowing the cancer host to stay in their own home is a great gift to them. But it does come at a price – and that must be recognised. It may even be that to care for your loved one you have put your entire life on hold in order to move in with them and help.

My sister did this. She left her college course in order to move in with my parents, and help with my mother's care. For her, it was a better option than being at a distance and unable to help – but you could never call it an easy choice.

It is possible that you may underestimate at the beginning what is involved in caring for someone who is very ill. Will changes need to be made to the house? Will they need a stairlift, or to have a bedroom made up downstairs. Do they have easy access to a bathroom, or are they unable to use those facilities anyway? When someone is ill, their needs are unlikely to stop during bedtime hours, so you may be on 24-hour call, 7 days a week. Is this realistic for you, or can you share the load in some way? Consider your own health – is it robust enough to deal with the demands that full-time caring will make on you?

When my grandfather became a carer for my grandmother, there was a great cost to his own health, even though my aunt and my mother went in regularly to help. So much so, in fact, that he died of heart failure and my grandmother had to go into residential care anyway. It is not worth making yourself ill in order to fulfil an obligation to your loved one, and no one should ask that of you. In fact you don't have a duty to give up your life to ease another's agony. If you do, please be aware that it is a choice.

What other choices are there, and how do you decide? For the very ill, there is hospital care – though standards vary and you may not be comfortable leaving your loved one in a medical facility if there is any other choice. Many hospices also have in-patient facilities, and can often deal with quite high medical care needs.

Far from the image that many have of depressing places where people go to die, the hospices I have visited have all been modern, airy, spacious and peaceful places. They are places where you would be pleased to go for afternoon tea, or a therapy treatment. The cancer host may be able to be cared for in such a place – either for the duration of their illness, or just for what is known as respite care. My mother stayed for a couple of weeks in a hospice for just such a respite. It wasn't her favourite time, as she preferred home, but it gave my father a much-needed break. Dad was able to fulfil one of his outside interests. He took part in a Shakespearean production at an open-air theatre near his home. How I enjoyed going to watch him (even though it rained). It was great to know he had a short time where he was doing something for himself.

If you do care for the cancer host at home, then get whatever help you can. We could not have managed in the later stages without the Macmillan nurses who came in to care for my mother. Their experience, caring natures, and calm acceptance of the situation made so much difference.

Being Told it's 'Terminal'

There are two different scenarios in which you may be 'told it's terminal'. One is sort of by default, where the cancer is diagnosed but no treatment to cure is offered. The second is where much treatment has been tried, but it turns out to have been a losing battle, or where time has allowed the cancer to grow and damage the body beyond repair. At this point there is no further purpose in trying to get rid of the cancer. These two scenarios are in fact very different.

The first is the situation we found ourselves in when my mother was diagnosed with secondary brain tumours. Even then, I'm not sure anyone really spelled out at the beginning that this meant she was likely to die. That's just not what they say. In any case the medical staff would certainly not have been able at that stage to answer the next big question – how long do we have together?

In fact they would have been as well not to answer. My friend's sister, Fern, was also in this kind of situation. She was diagnosed, after much uncertainty and pain, with a tumour on her spine. Fern was told that the hospital could offer treatment, but it would only prolong her life for a short time. (The original projection for her life was two weeks.) Fern's reaction was to *demand* the treatment – and she did the rest. She got better, raised her children and is still healthy today, over 20 years later.

This is why doctors are often reluctant to make predictions, because they know how easily they could be wrong. So even though it is frustrating not to have a crystal ball, you should regard this as a good thing. The uncertainty means that there are still possibilities - your loved one isn't gone just because someone handed them a diagnosis. The uncertainty works in your favour.

The second scenario is more like the situation we were in when the Macmillan nurses finally said to my father and me, "You do know she will die very soon, now, don't you?" Although of course we were not glad to lose her, there was a great feeling of relief. Finally someone had given us an indication of how much longer it would be. They were able to let us know that she would be gone in days rather than weeks, and in fact she lived about a week and a half after that day.

This may seem late to get some kind of a timescale, but I'm afraid that is the nature of the human body. It's unpredictable, because the thoughts of the person living inside it determine so much of how it lives, and fades. There are people like Fern who simply won't be told they're going to die, and others who are expected to live for a few months, but slip away within weeks.

It is likely that you will not find out that you are in this second type of scene until the end is close at hand. Don't be shocked and horrified if either you or others (including the cancer host) seem relieved. Being ill with cancer, or supporting someone else who is, can be just plain exhausting. If you're told you can't win, then it can be very peaceful to accept that this phase of life is ending, whether it's your body that's going to die or another's.

If you reach this time it would be a good idea to visit www.hospiceoftheheart.org, and to talk to those who can ease your loved one's passing. You can visit Chapter 9 to begin exploring the implications of the loss you are now facing.

Learn Calming Techniques

If you haven't done so already, the times when the going seems tough are good ones to introduce extra calming techniques into your life. You are probably holding an immense amount of physical tension in your body. You need to find ways to release it so that you don't suffer ill effects.

Calming techniques vary widely, but all serve the same purpose. You could read the book *Calm For Life* by Paul Wilson. It will help you to find a practical technique that particularly suits you. If you need something more direct and personal, you could join a meditation group or use a meditation CD. Yoga is also very beneficial, or there may be specific relaxation classes local to you. The Sedona Method (described in Chapter 6) is also very calming, as is sitting or walking in a garden or park. Many people have shrunk their problems to a manageable size whilst tramping out on a long hike.

After learning these techniques, the next step is remembering to use them! I was good at using relaxation techniques and visualisation when I was giving birth and had nothing else to do, but when my kids are pushing my buttons my relaxation techniques are the last thing on my mind.

It may help to set aside a specific time each day for some calming time for you. Make it an appointment with yourself, just as you learned in Chapter 5. The more you practise the technique you have chosen in your own time, the easier it will come to hand when you most need it.

Don't Suffer Alone

"A problem shared is a problem halved", the old saying goes. There is a lot of truth in that! When you are suffering alone, the chances are that you will feel much worse. The problems that you have will grow into impossible challenges, and you may despair of how you are going to deal with them. You may find that one reason why you are choosing to suffer alone is fear. If you are afraid to feel your emotions fully, this may make you hold back from sharing them with others.

To overcome this, you can make a conscious decision to dive into the centre of the emotion. All too often we believe that if we give in to a feeling it will conquer us. We have been taught that we need to control our emotions – think Spock in *Star Trek*, or the stiff upper lip of us Brits. In fact the truth is almost the opposite. If you dive into the emotion, let it wash over you, you often find that at the centre there is nothing there. It is a little like the eye of the hurricane. At the centre of even the strongest emotion there is a patch of calm, where the feeling is quieter even though it may still be there. So the fear that stops you from allowing your emotions to flow is keeping those emotions in the forefront of your mind. You can do this process of diving into the emotion very easily. All it takes is a quiet moment – on your own or with someone else. The emotion is absolutely *desperate* to be felt. All you have to do is loosen your chokehold on it for long enough to do that. If it makes you cry, then cry. If you feel the need to shout then do that too. The people around you will get over it.

Now you have handled your fear of how you feel, you are free to connect with others. They could be other friends or relatives of the cancer host, with whom you can share empathy and support. They could be other people whom you care about and who care about what's happening to you. They could be anyone who already qualified to be your emotional sounding board. You could get some Guatemalan Worry Dolls and tell your troubles to them. Or you could go deeper and say that you will share your feelings with God, the universe or the angels if that is your preference.

Find Your Inner Reserves

How do you react when faced with hard times? Do you crumble under pressure, or dig deep to find a way to keep going? Often it depends on whether you have enough of a reason. Parents find amazing reserves for their children. Whether it be cleaning up sick in the dead of night, or lifting a car off their injured child, the WHY of looking after a being that is so dear to them overcomes any obstacles.

You may have heard some wonderful tales of people overcoming great odds. For instance Joe Simpson who made it out of the Andes in spite of terrible injuries (his true story is told in the book and film *Touching The Void*). Another example is Immaculée Ilibagiza, who teaches forgiveness for those who carried out the atrocities in Rwanda (and killed most of her family) in her book *Left To Tell*.

Maybe you think these people are somehow special, or different from you. Well they're not. Yes, they have done amazing things, whether physical or emotional. But they have done them from resources we all have available to us. They did them because something drove them to extreme lengths, to find the reserves they needed.

You also have access to those reserves, so what is *your* reason?

What WHY is big enough for *you* to access that strength of character? If you're not convinced you really can tap into such reserves of strength, why not try borrowing them from someone else. Choose someone you admire, someone who has faced the sort of tests you are enduring, or a test you consider even harder. The person you first thought of is the right one. Then decide you're going to borrow their mental and emotional attitude for a while. You don't need to get in touch with them, just behave the way you believe they would. The truth is that we are all connected in some way, so you can 'borrow' strength from others.

Once you have tapped into your reserves (or borrowed them from someone else), simply keep taking one step at a time. As Lao-Tzu said, "A journey of a thousand miles must begin with a single step." Don't concern yourself with how you will cope with tomorrow, simply live through what you must today – and if you can manage to do it with a smile, so much the better.

Loss of the 'Person'

One of the tough times on your journey may come when you feel you have already lost the person you loved even though they are physically still present. This may happen by degrees. At a very early stage, as I have already mentioned, the cancer host's personality can change because of the challenges they are facing. The full personality that you loved isn't there just now. This could be temporary, or come and go as they respond to treatments and challenges that they face. It could also be part of a progression, a gradual loss of the person you knew. I felt this with my mother. It seemed that the happy side of her personality was eaten away. The part of Mum which always saw the problems, the one she had worked so hard to keep in check, gradually won the day. But that wasn't my *real* Mum.

At a later stage, you may feel there is nothing left of the person you knew. It may be very hard to continue caring for them if you feel this way. At this point it is especially important to remember the real them – and hold that 'them' true for you as you care for their physical self. If you can do this, you will be able to overlook the tougher parts of their exchanges with you. You can forgive them their present faults if you keep in mind that the real them would not be this way. It is a way of honouring the person you loved.

This is not to say that you should put yourself in any danger. If someone's personality has changed so much that they are a threat to you, then you absolutely must get help. However much you love them, it is not acceptable for you to be mistreated.

If the 'real them' appears in flashes, then fades away, try not to resent that. My colleague Nayna, whose father had Alzheimer's disease, found his moments of clarity the hardest times of all. But you can focus on the momentary gain, rather than what it shows you have lost.

Of course, the disappearance of the person you knew also means the loss of your relationship with them. If they are not really there, your relationship will change from one of equality to an almost parental, caring role. This may trigger your grief, so acknowledge it, and allow your grieving to begin. Grief is a process that allows us to adjust to new realities, and you will find it covered in more depth in Chapter 9.

Taking Difficult Decisions

There may be times during your loved one's treatment when you are asked to make some difficult decisions. Should they even be told they have cancer – particularly if they are either very young or elderly and confused? Should the cancer host be resuscitated if they have a heart attack? Nobody wants to be put in the position of making this sort of decision, but it is possible that this may fall to you. How do you handle it? Ideally you won't have to do it on your own. If you can discuss the matter with others who are affected, it should be easier to make the decision, unless there is a real difference of opinion.

First of all it's important to look at what is the 'default position'. What is being done while the decision is being made? In the examples I gave above, the default would probably be not to tell them in the first, and to resuscitate them in the second.

My view (as you probably realise), is that wherever possible the cancer host should be the one to make the decision, though there is nothing wrong with a supportive family discussion. This means that even if the medical team is worried about telling your loved one something about their condition, you at least talk over the subject with the cancer host. If they really don't want to know, they will probably change the subject or just plain not hear you – and then they will have made that decision. But if the cancer host wants to know, then they have a right to.

Many people have been told they were dying, and used this as an opportunity to find a sense of peace – possibly one that has escaped them all their life. Why deny them that? You won't go far wrong if you stick to the principle you've been using already of talking things through and accepting that the cancer host is the master of their own ship.

Audrey Jenkinson, in her book *Past Caring*, describes how her mother expressed quite definitely that she did not want to be kept alive, or resuscitated. She was perfectly able to make that decision even though communicating it was difficult. It proved hard to honour that request, as medical staff will always try to revive someone unless they know expressly not to.

In reality this means that when someone is admitted to hospital as an emergency, there will be no time to take ethical decisions. One person at death's door looks much like another and the emergency team will not have the information they need unless they are given it. So if your loved one has expressed their wish to go out gracefully, you will need to make sure *everyone* knows. It may mean you have to be with them on your own when they die, if you are caring for them at home.

If your loved one has gone past the point of being able to make their own decisions, and it is just a matter of time, don't be afraid to talk over what treatment they are being given with their medical team. Keeping their body in this world as long as possible is the remit we have given to our health services, but it may no longer be the approach that serves this person best. Of course, in order to take these or other difficult decisions, you have to be prepared to let your loved one go.

Let the Love In

When you can't change the reality of the circumstances, when everything has gone against you and the cancer host, when you are left only with the option of changing yourself, as Viktor Frankl said: how do you do that? One tool for doing that is allowing yourself to feel loved.

A client wrote on the form she sends in preparation for her coaching session recently, "I feel special and appreciated and loved at the moment." Is she any more special than last time we spoke? Any more loved? No! All that has happened is that she has let it in. She always was loved. She always was special, and probably people appreciated her even if they didn't always say so. The same is true for you.

You are loved, if you allow yourself to be. Just do a good deed, spare a thought or a smile for someone and you will get appreciation. The more open and loving you are, the more those things will be reflected back to you. So when I called this section Let the Love In, perhaps it should have been Let the Love Out! Even if you feel completely numb, that is just a defence against feeling the love you have, and the pain you have decided goes with that.

Transformation through Suffering

There is a process by which transformations are made. Take the example of oil. Trees become buried beneath the ground. Naturally they would form into peat if they were in a wet environment. Peat can be dried out and burnt as fuel, or used to add organic matter to other soils. But what happens if those trees become buried deep under the ground? Another factor comes into play. That factor is *pressure*. When great pressure is applied over a long time, the organic matter that makes up the trees is totally transformed and becomes oil. This is a completely different substance from the natural peat, and has some special properties, which we have been busy making use of in our modern society.

The same principle also applies to people. I watched a programme on the television last week about a particular raid on a German naval base in France during World War II. What was interesting to me was the description of how they trained the commandos for the raid; they used the same methods they do to train elite soldiers today. The main factor was to put the soldiers in situations beyond what they believed they could possibly handle. This is the origin of the modern assault course. Getting through those situations, surviving the tough regime, gave the soldiers the feeling that they could achieve anything! In other words the instructors applied PRESSURE, and the recruits underwent a transformation. As a result they showed extreme bravery as they carried out their (ultimately successful) raid. The Germans could not believe they would mount an assault on such a heavily defended base, and had great respect for these soldiers.

There are other forms of training that also use this principle. One example is Peak Potentials' *Enlightened Warrior Training Camp*, which I attended; I chose to put myself under that pressure voluntarily. The same applies to the exposure therapy that is used so successfully to overcome deeply held phobias. The pressure of being in contact with the object of the phobia transforms the person and their view of that object. It also explains the popularity of the (in my eyes) bizarre sport of bungee jumping. Once you have been able to take that step over the edge, what else might you be capable of?

What is the point of all this? Well, you're the one under pressure now. I don't believe that suffering is a good thing, or that we should seek it out. But I do believe the pressure it applies can be used for good. For now, just know that you won't come out the other end unchanged. But also know that the transformation will bring you closer to your true self than you have ever been, if you only let it.

ACTION STEP

Make a list of all the people you love, or have loved, in your life. Then add all the pets, places, houses, cars, or experiences you have loved. Write them all down. Feel the love you have for those things, and revel in it. Let the love out, then relax and know it has already come back.

8

ARRIVING PART 1 – REMISSION

At last, here it is. You've arrived at your destination. Your loved one has been given a clean bill of health. Not only is there light at the end of the tunnel, but you've made it out into that light. You could be tempted to think that the tunnel is behind you and that's the end of the story. But after all you've been through on your journey so far, it would be a shame not to take a few more steps. That will give you a chance to make the most of what you can gain from having made the journey.

Your Destination – Success

How do you feel about your loved one's recovery? Are you jubilant, or do you feel strangely numb? You may be overjoyed, or feel dead inside and wonder what's wrong with you. When a large part of your life has been focused on someone else's illness and that's gone, you can have mixed feelings. On the one hand it's great that the cancer isn't hanging over you all, but on the other there is now a gap in your life. If it is this way for you, don't worry about it. Just as it takes time to adjust to a new reality after diagnosis, it can also do so now. It's like you've worn a rut in your mind on a path that says "my friend/relative has cancer". That path of thought is now a habit. Like all habits, you can change it, but it will take time.

One way to change that habit is to make sure you mark this occasion. It's not enough to visit the hospital and be told 'the scan was clear' – or even more distantly, to hear about it on the phone. It's important to celebrate this new phase and the hope for the future it brings.

If you're close to the cancer host (who of course isn't hosting anything any more), you may want to do this with them. Your loved one may want to throw a 'recovery party', and if so I hope you join in with gusto. On the other hand they may feel that it's tempting fate; that if they count on their health then somehow it will be more likely to be taken away from them. In this case I hope that your loved one is at least able to feel grateful that they have made it to this point, as that feeling of gratitude will help them.

So what do you do if your loved one just wants to ignore the whole issue of cancer or remission – pretend it never happened? Well, you could always celebrate by yourself. Raise a glass to them, and toast their future health. Or you could create some kind of a ritual – perhaps laying your Cancer Success Plan away (or even burning it), with thanks for the support it gave you.

Maybe the thought of burning your Plan terrifies you. What if the cancer comes back? Is this what you are secretly expecting? If so, take a good long look at where that thought is coming from. Address your deepest fears using the skills you have learned. My belief is that the Plan has done its work and you should let it go. If you were to face another journey with cancer, you would create a new one anyway. Your definition of success, your starting point and your inner self would all be different. You could find the same resources again if you needed to, anyway – after all you now know where to look.

Another way to mark the passing of the time of cancer in your loved one's life, would be to write about what this stage means to you in your journal.

You Can Never Return to Where You Set Off

Whilst you are in the midst of your journey with cancer, you have the hope that once your loved one gets the 'all clear', everything will get back to normal. Life will be just like it was before. The trouble is that the 'normal' you knew is really gone.

For one thing, your loved one is not exactly the same person they were before they had cancer. They may have changed a lot, both physically and emotionally. Also, the purpose of this book was to help you change yourself – in the best possible way, for your greater good and empowerment. So you're not the same person you were either.

Where does that leave the old 'normal'? Probably long gone. The place you started from was a place of innocence, of not knowing what you had to face ahead of you. You cannot reclaim that innocence. What you can claim is something better. If you can be fully at peace with all that has happened, if you can even be glad that you had the chance to take this journey, then you will see your destination with new eyes. You really can find this place to be somewhere better than where you were before.

One point of view you could use is that you *have* in fact returned to where you started, but it is your view of that place that is different. T.S Eliot wrote in *Four Quartets*:

> We shall not cease from exploration
> And the end of all our exploring
> Will be to return to where we started
> And know the place for the first time

You can find a modern parable for this type of journey in *The Alchemist* by Paulo Coelho, a novel that I highly recommend.

Everyone is Changed by the Experience

What kind of changes can you expect in yourself and others who have been on their own journey? To start with, you may all be exhausted. Absolutely physically and mentally drained by the whole experience. This will be less so if you have been making sure to take care of yourself, but it is a common feeling. All the energy you have been putting into supporting others, and into worrying about the outcome, could have wearied you. You may not even realise just how much tension you have been holding in your body until it's gone. Exhaustion can be a feature of life after cancer for a little while.

Some may feel they have lost confidence, and this may also be something you find in the person who has overcome the cancer. It may have shaken their personal belief – or on the other hand it could have strengthened it greatly. Imagine knowing you conquered a disease that everybody fears so much! Your loved one's attitude to life may also have changed. Were they happy-go-lucky before, but are now more fearful for the future? Did they previously dwell on possible disasters, but now are just determined to get the most from every moment they have? Everyone's reaction is slightly different, and yours will be as well.

One change I hope you will see in those around you is a new depth of wisdom. The journey you have all taken has given you the chance to tap into depths most people hardly even know are there. If you see growth in others around you, you can be sure you will also find that growth in yourself.

You may also find you have a whole new set of values. Your idea of what is truly important in life could be very different from what it was at the start of your journey. Perhaps you have even discovered those values for the first time. This is great! It means you can now measure every decision you make about the direction of your life, or how you choose to spend your time, against your new values to see if it fits. You will then live your life with much more intention and purpose than most, and it will bring you joy.

Are They Cured?

Cancer is so tricky, isn't it? We all know that nobody ever says "You're cured" to someone who has had cancer. When new drugs are tested the statistics that are used to decide whether it was a success are not 'numbers of people cured, they are 'years of survival', or even the 'extra time' that a person survives on one regime of treatment as opposed to another.

Many people write about the politics of cancer, and they call into question this way of determining success or failure; can it really be a success to increase someone's survival for just a few months? I'm sure you probably have your own strong opinions by now. What all this means to you and your loved one is that you won't get a person in a white coat saying that your loved one is cured. Remission is a 'wait and see' game. There will almost certainly be future monitoring involved. Each scan will be something to be nervous about, and if each one is clear then gradually your loved one may become more optimistic about the future.

Some people definitely *are* cured. Not only has the particular tumour or tumours completely disappeared, but either all the remaining cancer cells have been destroyed, or their body has re-learned to deal with them. I say re-learned because cancerous cells crop up in all our bodies – they are like a faulty copy from one cell to another. Our immune systems have ways to recognise them and get rid of them before they do any harm. Normally, it's nothing to worry about, so don't make it into something to fear. Cancer becomes a problem when that system breaks down. So when your loved one's immune system gets going again, it can protect them from cancer returning in the future. Nobody can tell you whether your loved one is one of those who are cured - those like Fern in the last chapter who, far from having two weeks to live, went on to a long and healthy life.

The worst problem is when you, or they, have an expectation

or a fear of the cancer returning. This can cloud your feelings and make it hard to just get on and enjoy life. Far better to take what you have learned and use it to encourage you to make the most of every single day from now on.

Re-Evaluate What is Important

Now it's time to take stock. What did you learn from this experience? It may have been a short journey or a long one. What are you bringing from that journey to the rest of your life? It is possible that you might need to take some time out from your life to fully process what you have gone through. Of course you will have been working on this as you went through your journey, with the help of this book, but now you will begin to get some benefit from hindsight. It can be difficult to see the bigger picture when you are still taking one step at a time on your journey.

Now you can look back. Here are some questions you might want to consider as you do so:

- What has this experience taught you? What have you learned about yourself, your relationships and your purpose in life?
- How can you apply what you have learned to your life now, and as you move forward?
- What is the most important area in which you want to make changes?
- What difference has the experience made to your religion or spirituality, if any?

- What is the one thing you need to do to make this journey have meaning for you? (If you don't have any ideas about this right now, read Chapter 11 and see if it inspires you).

The Crisis is Over – What Needs to Change?

Having answered the questions in the section before, you may have a pretty good idea of some things you want to change in your life. You won't rush in and change everything at once, but this is the time to start turning your life towards the direction you want it to go. We all deserve to be happy, and it's up to you to take the steps to make your life fit in with your happiness. You will never find happiness from outside sources, be they riches or relaxation. It comes from inside. But if you make your life fit you better then it will be easier to find that happiness inside.

It is time to start planning (again). But this time you have a blank canvas – you can take your life in any direction you want, as long as you stay true to your values. You could use the Wheel of Life chart from Chapter 4.

Other ways to find out what you want are to create a dream board or to write a list containing 101 intentions. Both fulfil the same purpose, so use the one that suits you best. You could even do the writing first, and then make a dream board for the goals you are pursuing now. A dream board is simply a large board where you pin or paste pictures or words which represent your ideal life. What has to be there for your life to truly represent the deeper you? If you prefer you can use a book, but then you need to remember to open it often.

The 101 intentions process is also simple. Write the numbers from 1 to 101 on separate lines and then fill in the blanks. Write everything you would like to BE, DO or HAVE in your life. This could range from BE peaceful, GO snowboarding, to HAVE a Maserati Spyder; or from BE a concert pianist, DANCE the Macarena, to HAVE time freedom. Some areas for improvement in your life that you might like to consider include these:

- Looking after and making time for yourself.

- Loving the people around you *as they are.*

- Making your work fit with your life purpose, so it is something you love to do and doesn't need to be balanced out so much. (I think those who make much of work/life balance do so in the assumption that you don't enjoy your work, or feel fulfilled by it.)

- If you can't achieve the last point, or until you do, keeping a good balance between work and social activities.

- Improving your living environment.

- Recreation – making sure you indulge in activities that re-create you on a regular basis.

Giving Thanks and Feeling Gratitude

As well as looking at what needs to change in your life, there is another side of the coin. This is the side where you feel grateful for *what you already have.* However much there is to change in your life, there will also be some things you can feel grateful for. You don't think so? Well you could start as I mentioned already with being grateful for your loved one's health. How about being grateful for your own health, and that of anyone else that you love.

You had enough money to buy this book, or were able to borrow it from the library. You have eyes to read or ears to hear the book read to you. The message is that you can always find something to be grateful for – especially if you consider what it would be like to lose those things.

Once you have got in touch with that feeling of gratitude, it is important to acknowledge it in some way. You could write a list of what you are grateful for. You could give money, or your time, to a charity (especially if there is a group which has been of great help recently, and as long as it doesn't keep you thinking about cancer too much). You could write a letter of thanks or a poem for someone who has helped you or your loved one. I'm sure you can think of many more ways.

Above all else, take time to recognise the gratitude you feel for your loved one's recovery. You now have the opportunity to spend more time together, address any remaining issues with your relationship, and appreciate the fact that they are still around!

Where is Your Relationship Now?

Any relationship you are in could have been changed as a result of your journey, but I am talking mainly about your relationship with the person who had the cancer. Their illness may have put your relationship under strain and stress (or perhaps it was already under stress before). You may have felt a sense of duty towards this person during their illness, or the old balance of energy between you could have shifted as they needed more help.

Once the cancer is gone, where does that leave your

relationship now? It would be nice to think that this experience will have brought you closer together, but sadly this is not always the case. For one thing, you can only deliver your side of the relationship. If your loved one has withdrawn from you then you can't control that. Alternatively you may be harbouring some resentment towards them, either because of the way they've behaved or else just because of the attention they've been getting.

All the methods you have learned on your Inner Journey will be of help to you now in dealing with the emotions surrounding your relationship. Your newfound communication skills are also there; now the cancer is less in the way, you may be able to talk more freely. Perhaps you could share your hopes and dreams for the future, and talk over what you both learned. This experience might act as a catalyst to allow you to let go of old issues, mend fences and dissolve any petty disagreements.

However, what if you feel your relationship is completely in tatters? For instance, what if you chose to stay with your partner whilst they had cancer because you felt a sense of duty? Well, if that's so then congratulations – you have done a very selfless thing. If you feel that your duty has now come to an end and you're thinking of leaving them, I would recommend you don't do anything too hasty. At this point in time your emotions are very raw. You (and they) have been through a lot. It will take a little time to get to know the new them, and the new you.

The first step is to deal with your own life and your own issues. Go through the process above and really consider what you can improve about your life. Don't ditch the relationship you have until you know for sure you've done everything you can to save it.

Over many months, my friend Amalia often told me that she was having problems in her marriage. It was hard to understand because her husband seemed such a lovely man. Then I spoke to her again a couple of months later, and everything had changed. She had found a job she loved, was feeling altogether better about life, and her husband was being fabulous! She was happier generally, and her marriage got better as a result. Your journey and its outcome could well have similar results

Take your time. Deal with your own situation and work on your own happiness. Let your loved one know what you want in your life, and what you are working towards. Love this person as they are now, because they are who they are. As author Stephen Covey says in his book *The 8th Habit*, "love is a verb" – you have to *be loving* to really have love. If your relationship can't be mended, then this will become clear in time. There is no need to rush into anything.

Relating to 'Outsiders'

There may be some people in your life who really don't understand what you've been through. In fact, I'm sure there will be. Some will appear to think that now your loved one is better you should 'pull your socks up' and get back to normal. After all, from their point of view, the problem is over. Why should you still be affected? Please forgive them for their ignorance. If they have never been on a journey like yours, how can they possibly know what's involved? It's similar to the way that no one can explain what it is like to be a parent; you only get that knowledge from personal experience. 'Outsiders' can't possibly know how you feel (even if they say they do).

Only you know how long it will take you to process what you have been through. You probably won't know yourself until it's happened, as well. Of course you also know that you won't be getting back to exactly where you were before anyway. The new you may have different priorities, and this often has an effect on others. If your experience makes you feel a great urge to spend six months on an ashram in India, your friends are likely to notice that you're not there! But that's your business, not theirs. Just understand that they can't understand. Tell them how you feel and about your decisions. They will have to accept that it is up to you.

Tell the people around you if you still need their support, or find others who do have some idea of what you are going through. You might choose to keep in touch with people you have met through local support groups or forums even if you don't need to spend so much time in those places now – just because they saw how you've been forged in the fire on your journey.

Above all, never ask someone's permission to do the things you choose to do. Only ask him or her to support you. You are in control of your own destiny.

Rebuilding Strength

All of the practical and emotional impacts we looked at in the previous chapters will have had an effect on you. The physical results of the stress you have been under may be immense. This will be true for the person who had cancer as well, especially if they had conventional treatments such as chemotherapy or radiotherapy. There may also be a mental exhaustion from so much feeling – such intensity of emotion that you're not used to. Now you need to take time to recuperate.

If at all possible, it would be good to get away from your day-to-day life. Take a holiday, or go on a retreat. This could be just a few days, or a longer break. What you will need depends on what your own level of exhaustion is. Allow your body to react to the tension you have been feeling and can now release.

If you can't get away, then keep your commitments to the minimum you can for a while and rest at home. You may even find you get ill at this time if you have been using great inner strength to keep going against all the odds. Sometimes this is just the body's way of getting you to rest! After a time of resting, you will be ready to begin strengthening through exercise, both physical and emotional. For both you need to start gradually, and build up as you go, especially if you haven't been exercising regularly so far.

Physical exercise could start with walking, swimming, or even just a little stretching. Emotionally the exercise is the same as the Inner Journey. Continue (or start) to keep a journal; join a meditation group; seek counselling or life coaching if you are finding it difficult to make sense of the experience. You will become emotionally stronger if you spend time with your feelings and allow them to pass through you, without holding on to them.

Live in Hope, Not Fear

It is understandable, with the unpredictable nature of cancer, to fear for your loved one's health in the future. Of course I've been suggesting that you acknowledge your fears and deal with them. But if you find yourself feeling fearful for your loved one's health a lot, and for a long time, then there is something that needs to be done.

It is important that you find a way to let that fear go. Worry has been described as being like negative prayer. Every time your mind plays out the scene of what you fear might happen, it is as though you *wanted* that to happen. Your conscious mind knows that you really want to avoid that outcome, but your subconscious mind doesn't know that. You are effectively taking the cancer, which happened in the past, and dragging it into the present with you. Why would you want to do that? Let it stay in the past where it belongs.

How do you make sure you are living in hope? Ideally you notice when you're not, let go of the underlying fear, and replace the negative visions with positive ones. If you find yourself thinking, "I hope the cancer doesn't come back", replace that with a vision of your loved one looking healthy and active. If you have something planned in the future such as a holiday or a family get-together, you could picture them there, and this will help you to feel more positive. This isn't about making your loved one healthier – it's about you feeling better. At the same time, your increased confidence in their health may just give them a boost.

After my mother-in-law's treatment, she was feeling very tired and said to me that she was beginning to feel her age. A morning's shopping would completely wear her out. I told her I was sure it was just an after-effect of the chemotherapy, which would pass in time. And it has. She has now moved to live near us, and you will find her on the seafront most days, rain or shine: she even goes to the shops in her hiking boots so she can walk on the beach before she goes home.

Confidence in the Future

No one can tell you what the future holds. Some of that depends on you, some on your loved one and some on what fate brings. As you have no idea what's going to happen, you might as well stay positive.

Allow the experience you have been through to sharpen your focus in the present. Plan for the future, and let go of the past. Throw off any temptation to feel bad about what has happened or worry about what's to come. You don't have time for that, because the rest of your life is waiting.

ACTION STEP

Create a ceremony to celebrate the return to health of the person who had cancer. This could be anything from a party to a symbolic burning of something relating to the time when they had cancer. Put the cancer in the past where it belongs.

9

ARRIVING PART 2 - ADJUSTING
TO LOSS

We have already covered one possible destination for your journey: recovery or remission for your loved one. But there is another possibility - that you will be bereaved. The word itself is emotive, suggesting that something has been torn from you.

Your partner, relative or friend has found that there is no possibility for them of recovering from their cancer, and so their time here is at an end. It may well feel as if your life is ending also. As in every life event there are as many different reactions as there are people, and yet there are some common themes.

You can also choose how you look at the situation you are facing; there are more and less helpful attitudes you can take.

Accept That They Are OK

Your first task is just this – to accept that the ending of life is fine for that person. Whatever your beliefs about an afterlife, the suffering of the person's body ends at the point of death. It must! Cancer has weakened the body to the point at which it no longer works. This means that the physical pain or trauma is now finished. They are now free.

It is tempting to feel that your loved one has 'lost' the life they might otherwise have had. As a society we mourn especially hard when someone dies in their youth. We are upset that they never married, had children, got a job, a fast car and so on. I believe they have lost nothing. Those things were never guaranteed for anyone. Not one thing has been lost, and there is only meaning for you in focusing on the experiences they *did* have in their life.

Children seem to find this easier to accept than adults. Often when they are diagnosed with terminal illnesses, children focus on the love they have experienced in their lives. They have not become attached to experiences of which really they know nothing. We have a lot to learn from the way they focus on the present rather than the future.

So, accepting this fact, it then follows that grief is actually about the people left behind. It is a self-centred emotion. This is not criticising the feeling, merely telling the truth about it. When we are feeling grief we are effectively saying – "they SHOULD still be here with me. I want it!"

The eighteenth-century mystic Swedenborg described his visions of spirits passing into the next world, and their desire to comfort those left behind. "It's all right, I'm fine now" they try to communicate. This might indeed comfort those left behind, but these spirits are missing some of the point. The grief stems from a perceived gap in your life – a gaping hole where such a short time ago was a living, breathing person.

The Beauty of Preparedness

I don't think anyone can ever truly prepare for the death of a loved one. Just as no one can explain to you how it will feel to become a mother – you wouldn't understand however hard they may try. So it is impossible to imagine how the world will feel without that person in it. There is something different, though, when you know someone has cancer. Right from the point of diagnosis, there it is on the table. Even if it isn't discussed (and if you've been reading this book so far, I hope it has been), there is always the possibility of death lurking in the shadows.

In some cases of cancer, diagnosis comes at a very late stage, the disease progresses swiftly and death comes soon. A more common scenario is of hopes raised, progress and setbacks - a roller coaster ride. It may not seem so, but this can be a blessing. When a person dies suddenly, for example of a heart attack or accident, in addition to all the other emotions there is a terrible sense of shock.

One lady I knew closely, Maria, was only a few months from retirement when she died suddenly on Christmas Eve. She felt a little unwell in the morning, went to bed and was gone by the afternoon. Not one member of the family had even realised she was ill. The numbness and unreality of the situation were beyond belief.

In contrast, when you know someone has cancer, opportunities open up. You will already have addressed unfinished business in both practical matters and relationships – assuming you all chose to take that opportunity. This is why it is so important to face up to the possibility of death at an early stage, deal with what seems important, then get on with the business of living. When you are at the stage of bereavement you then have the comfort of knowing that your loved one tackled the things that were important to them.

There may also be a point at which your loved one feels ready to go, having simply had enough of fighting. They may feel that whatever comes next must be better than this struggle to hang on to existence. Our job as helpers is to support that decision. How much better if your loved one is able to let go of life gently, rather than having it ripped from them.

It may be that you have the chance to say farewell to your loved one. This is not always the case. The ending of life does not follow some pre-set pattern. Some cling to life beyond what seems reasonable, others slip away unexpectedly.

In my own case with my mother, I knew she was dying. I left her for my final time a week before the end, and I knew it would be the last time I saw her alive. She was already 'sleeping' and not seemingly aware of me in the room. And still, saying 'goodbye' rather than 'see you soon' was the hardest thing I have had to do to this day. However prepared you are, saying goodbye can still be difficult. Not having that chance hurts too.

Not long after my mother died, my boyfriend James took me to a concert by Lou Reed. James had recently bought an album, entitled *Magic and Loss*. I hadn't really paid much attention to the songs, but when we got to the concert we were told that this would be a performance of the whole album. As I listened to the words it dawned on me that this was a story – a story of friends dying of cancer. As the tears streamed down my face, the concert came to a song called *No Chance*. Lou told of his frustration of expecting to make his regular visit, only to have his friend pass away suddenly during the week. "I never had the chance to say goodbye" he sang. "It doesn't make it easy when you do" I whispered to myself in the darkness of the auditorium. That was indeed a magical evening, which allowed much of my grief to flow. Now I can look back and see the comfort I have in being able to say that goodbye.

Only you can know what is right for you – if you do get to make the choice. If not then please just accept that there is no 'right' or better way. This is just the way it is for you this time.

It probably does help to be prepared for the physical reality of death. My mother-in-law was given a leaflet by the hospital when a close relative was dying, which gave some information about the process. It may seem absurd to need such a leaflet, but so few of us have seen someone die that it makes perfect sense. For instance, it is unlikely that your loved one will be conscious at the end, but they may respond to what is said to them at the time. Creating a calm and loving atmosphere may well soothe their passing. It may be helpful for you to wish them well on their journey and let them know you are happy for them to leave when they are ready.

I suggest you consult with those caring for your loved one. Ask them what to expect. If you want to include others at the moment of death, they will most likely do their best to accommodate those wishes.

Allowing Some Choice or Control

Life seems to throw challenges at us – and death especially feels like one of these. We may feel as though we have no control. The fight with cancer may have been long and difficult, and now it looks as if it is ending. However reluctant you (and they) may feel, it is possible to introduce some element of choice.

Here are a few things that together you may be able to influence:

- *Choosing the place*

    It may be possible to choose the place where this person makes their departure from physical life. If you have been able to care for them at home they may be able to die there also. This was the case for my mother. She disliked hospitals intensely, and I am sure that it made her final days much calmer to be at home. It may even be possible to move your loved one home when the end is near, if you so choose. On the other hand, the idea of your loved one dying in your house may fill you with horror. In this case you can explore the options of hospice or hospital, which will give you a much higher level of support. Neither is right or wrong, simply how you feel, and how you feel is important. It is not selfish to need more support at this time.

- *Choosing the time*

    You may feel that what you want most is to delay your loved one's death as much as possible. This seems to be the assumption that is made by default. And so it is likely that there will be medical intervention that will keep your loved one alive far beyond the point at which they would have died without it. This means that there may be some choice about lessening that intervention, or changing its nature from life-prolonging to more easing of symptoms. You may feel some reluctance to raise such a topic – perhaps it seems somehow wrong to ask for them to die sooner – but it may be a very helpful discussion to have. At best, your loved one will be able to express that they have had enough, and no longer want to be kept alive. I have a good friend who is a doctor, and she has had many such conversations with patients. The extreme is one gentleman, Trevor, whose life was being prolonged by treatment. However, his quality of life was deteriorating with time. He took the choice as to when his treatment would be withdrawn, effectively choosing his 'death day'. His family and friends gathered for a party on the ward and sent him off in style. What a way to go!

- *Choosing the atmosphere*

Planning a death in advance is not something that is often done in polite society – at least not in the culture I live in. But there is much that can be done to ease a departure from this life. This is probably the reason that traditionally a minister of religion would have been summoned to the person's deathbed. It was thought that they could absolve the person of their sins, so easing their passage to the next world. In the modern world, this would comfort few of us, although there are some for whom the closeness of death opens up ideas they thought were long buried! Your loved one may suddenly wish to talk about spiritual matters. They may begin to think over their fears or hopes about what may come next for them. Setting the atmosphere should involve thinking about this person's wishes. What would they find soothing? Massage, aromatherapy, music or healing can be a beneficial part of death. You could read a special poem to your loved one, or simply tell them all the wonderful things that having them in your life has brought.

In my view, the most important thing would be not to set a solemn mood. When death approaches, this is not the time to ask your loved one to fight or hang on to life. That time has passed. Celebrate their life, wish them well, and send them on their way.

Feelings of Relief or Guilt

When you have been looking after someone, or worrying about them, for a long time it is like being a stretched rubber band. The tension builds up as time goes on. With cancer, as many other illnesses, it can go on for a very long time. My mother was ill for eight months from diagnosis to her death, plus the time before she was diagnosed when we weren't sure what exactly was wrong. Though not a long time compared to some other conditions, the better part of a year is still a long time to have that uncertainty on your mind every day. It's a long time not to want to make too many plans, just to keep concentrating on another person. In relative terms eight months is quite a short journey even with cancer. For many there is treatment, remission, relapse and years of plain worry.

So when a loved one who has been suffering dies, is it any wonder that the first emotion many of us feel is relief? Relief for the deceased, that they are no longer suffering. And relief for yourself, that at last you have an ending – even if not the one you were hoping for. The tension on the rubber band is gone. You may almost have forgotten who you were without that tension. For those involved in physically caring for a dying friend or relative the relief may be immense. Even more immense than the burden you have been bearing. In fact the relief may be so strong that it seems to overpower the feelings of grief. When my mother died, I was relieved that the long drawn-out process was over for her, and also for my Dad and sister, who bore the brunt of the caring. What I found (and others have described the same thing) was that grief caught me by surprise, because I didn't expect to feel it as I was so relieved.

It hit me at the funeral. When the minister used Mum's favourite quote from the bible, "I will lift up mine eyes to the hills, from whence cometh my help", I felt she was there, and was also reminded that in a physical sense she never would be again.

There can also be a flip side to the relief: feelings of guilt. Guilt at feeling relieved. Guilt over what you said, or didn't. Guilt over how you cared for them. Guilt over how often you visited, or didn't. Guilt that you had wished they could die sooner because you were just *so* tired. There is only one way to handle these feelings of guilt – to acknowledge them, and then refuse to entertain them. They serve no possible purpose. You cannot, however much you may wish or visualise, undo one thing you have done or said. The answer to these feelings is to say to yourself whenever they come up, "Thank you very much, I was doing the best I could at the time". If you do this every time, the feelings will lessen as time goes by. As my father says, "You can only start from where you are now"!

Unfinished Business

I hope this book has encouraged you to deal with a lot of 'business' long before the point at which this person lets go of life. But it is almost certain that something will be left unsaid or undone. One of the hardest things is no longer being able to communicate with them, and so lacking a sense of completeness. At this point, you have to accept that what is left unfinished is now your responsibility, and yours alone. The solution is for you to attend to your side of this incomplete item.

One technique that could be helpful is writing a letter to the deceased. The important ground rule here is that it should be done for positive reasons. Not to get at the person you have lost, but to let go of past hurts or feelings unsaid, in order to move on. You can also use a letter to express all the positive things you wish you had said to your loved one. This can be done when a person has just died, or many years afterwards. The task is to write everything in the letter – don't edit or think too hard. Just pour the feelings onto the page, feeling the lightening of your load as you do so. Many people find it helpful to then burn or rip up the letter. You can say aloud, "I let go of these feelings so that I can move on with my life." Then do just that – move on.

This is a really important process, especially if you are holding any resentment towards the person. Negative feelings whirring round in your mind cause your body to create toxic substances. I once heard a quote which relates to this. Nelson Mandela said, "Resentment is like drinking poison and then hoping it will kill your enemies." If the object of your resentment is already dead, why are you still drinking the poison? If the unfinished business is something for which you are blaming yourself – you wish you had said or done something differently – then it is important for you to forgive yourself. The letter writing process may be helpful here also. If not, then every time you feel regret, make an effort to remember something positive about your relationship with that person. This way you will replace sadness with good memories as time goes by.

Stages of Grief

According to research conducted by psychiatrists J. Bowlby and C.M. Parkes, there are four stages of grief that people commonly experience. You may find that one or more of these phases describe where you are in your grief at any time. Your progression from one stage to another may not be smooth, and where you are can vary from day to day. The four stages are:

1. **Numbness**. This is where you may be in shock, feeling disbelief and cut off from reality.
2. **Yearning, pining**. Here you find you wish to bring back the person, long for them. You may feel much anger and disappointment at this stage.
3. **Depression, disorganisation and despair**. Now you find it difficult to function in your everyday life. You may struggle to concentrate or not be able to bear thinking about the future.
4. **Recovery and reorganisation**. At this stage more positive feelings begin to surface. You are ready to take the first steps of moving forward with your life, and adjusting to your new reality.

When you first reach the stage of recovery, it is likely to be fragile. You may start by catching fleeting glimpses of how life may be. It is tempting at this stage to slide back into guilt, thinking "How can I be thinking of the future when he or she is not here?" Guard against this temptation. Guilt serves no one, especially not your loved one, who has left already.

Describing these phases of grief makes them seem passive, as though you have no control over your route through them. There is a benefit to taking your time. No one can tell you how long it should take you to move from one stage to another. There are many things that affect your ability to adjust and move on through this unfamiliar landscape.

A more 'active' way of looking at grief comes from William Worden, who described a series of four tasks that are involved in mourning.

1. **To accept the reality of the loss**. This shows that you can make the choice to face this reality with courage, and resist the temptation to deny it.

2. **To experience the pain of grief**. This task is where you dive into the pain. When giving birth, a mother is encouraged to flow with the pain, rather than resisting it. If you give yourself the time and the space to do this with your grief, you will allow the emotions to flow rather than become stuck. Self-medicating with alcohol, or anything else that prevents you truly feeling your emotions, would be avoiding this task.

3. **To adjust to the environment where the deceased is missing**. The loss of someone close to you changes the scenery

of your every day. In fact the build up to death may have changed your life beyond recognition, so that it revolved around caring for the cancer host. When they die, this is a huge adjustment. Your task now is to create the new landscape of your life, metaphorically moving the furniture to at least partly fill the hole that they have left.

4.   **To emotionally relocate the deceased and move on**. This task involves making a space for your loved one as a memory rather than a current relationship. Keeping them in your heart in this way allows you to look forward to a future without them and not feel bad about yourself for doing so.

You will find a way through these phases and tasks. The human spirit is resourceful and resilient. In the early stages it may feel as though your world has ended. And so in a sense it has. However, there is a new world for you to step into, when you are ready.

Who Was This Person to You?

Grief is a variable emotion. It depends more on your relationship than on the person who has died. It stands to reason that your life will be changed more by losing a beloved pet that woke you every morning with an enthusiastic lick, than your Great Aunt Bertha to whom you were introduced once at the age of three.

Let's look at how that relationship will change your grief, depending on who the person you have lost was in your life. I have divided these into four main groups:

- Losing a partner
- Losing a parent
- Losing a sibling Or friend
- Losing a child

Losing a Partner

When your life partner dies, everything changes beyond recognition. Every space in your home reminds you of them. The majority of your activities outside of work may have involved them in some way. Even for activities that did not, you may still miss being able to report on them.

One everyday difference that continues into the years to come is that of having to do *everything*. There is no one else to put the bins out, feed the cat, use the washing machine or iron, put up a shelf, and make the dinner or the beds. Suddenly tasks that were someone else's responsibility become yours.

If yours has been a long relationship, you may not even remember how to do some of these things, and have to relearn. Of course, during the illness, you may have been taking on these additional tasks. This may have seemed temporary, though, and you may find it unwelcome having to shoulder these extra burdens for weeks, months and years ahead.

Another challenge on losing a partner is that of your social life. My lovely neighbour Patricia had to persuade her son to join the local golf club after his father died, in spite of the fact that he had never had the inclination to lift a club. The reason – it was one of those old-fashioned institutions where ladies could not be members in their own right, only with a man, either a husband, or in this case a son. My reaction was that I wouldn't want to be a member of such an institution, but for her it was a large part of her social life. Bad enough to lose a life partner, but to be excluded from the club as well would have been an additional blow.

Even without the rules of a straight-laced institution, this removal of a social life can happen. If you socialised as a couple, some of those opportunities are likely to disappear. It will be up to you to be as creative as Patricia in finding ways to put your social life back on track. This may seem to be the least of your concerns in the aftermath of bereavement, but as time goes by you will rebuild a better life if you are socially active.

As a couple you probably daydreamed of the future, talked and planned the way your life would be in times to come. We are all liable to build these castles in the air. Now those hopes and dreams are dashed. You probably had a list of things you were planning to do together, and now those things seem hollow. It is time for you to accept that your priorities may be different in the future. Some of your dreams may still come to pass. They will not be the same without your partner, and yet they may be more moving as a result.

Some dreams you will have to let go of now that your loved one is gone. Still, other dreams will appear as part of your new life. I hope you will take this experience you have been through and realise that life is too short to build castles in the air. They need to be on the ground, built and enjoyed now. I'm not saying you should never make plans for the future. Just resolve to take action to turn those dreams into reality sooner rather than 'one day' or never.

One final point to consider is that not every relationship is one hundred percent perfect (no, really). So there is the possibility that some elements of your life may actually improve now you are on your own. If your partner liked everything to be precise and you would prefer to leave the washing up in the sink (or vice versa), you may relish the freedom of no longer having to negotiate terms with someone else. If you find an element of enjoying new freedom creeping into your feelings, please accept that this is normal. Even the very best relationships involve some degree of compromise, and it is okay to appreciate your independence. Far from being disloyal, it is a sign that you are beginning to adjust successfully to the change you find in your life.

Losing a Parent

Death of a parent is very different from that of a partner. Rather than an equal, you have lost a person who (at least at some stage) was in a position of power in relation to you. This loss may have happened to some extent before your parent died. Often there is a degree of role reversal when someone is ill. You find yourself caring for your parent in ways they may once have done for you – especially if you are involved with nursing them. This creates a strange set of emotions. It feels wrong. They are *supposed* to be the strong one. I found that I had to block my awareness of this role reversal in order to cope with the situation.

After your parent has gone, you may also have lost a safety net, or be mourning the fact that you never had one. I remember saying to my best friend after my mother died that I had always had this unspoken assumption - if everything went wrong, if all else failed, I could always go home to Mum. For whatever reason that was related to my Mum and not my Dad, so it was now gone. It was really scary. No matter how unlikely that I would ever use it, my ultimate back-up plan was no more! Bless my friend, for she immediately said, "Well, if it ever happens, I'll take you in!"

A parent may also be a storehouse of information, advice and even recipes! I can no longer ask anyone what time I was born, how old when I cut my first tooth. (Well, I can ask, but my father can't remember.) When my children ask me these things I have to say "I don't know". Not especially important, but it's one of those little things you don't appreciate until it's gone. Just like the special cookies we enjoyed as children, which I could not find the recipe for in my mother's kitchen. Still, sometimes information comes back from the most unlikely sources. An old school friend whom I contacted through *Friends Reunited* turned out to have written down Mum's recipe for Jam Crater cookies – yum! I still miss her apple pie, though.

This sort of thing can apply whatever age you are when you lose your parent. But for those who lose a parent at a young age there are added challenges. You may feel you have had to grow up too soon. The person you were counting on to support you emotionally (or often financially) as you set off into the world is no longer there.

As with everything, there is much you can do in controlling your own response to the circumstances. I hope you will find the support you need from others. They may be people you would not have reached out to had things been different. Generally, people will be glad to be asked for help. You will also find reserves of strength in yourself that you did not know were there.

Again, as with losing a partner, there is also the need to let go of expected future experiences. For me this involved becoming a mother myself. I had expected to disagree with Mum about bringing up my children, but none the less expected her to be around in support. When I did have my first son seven years after my mother's death I was very glad of my mother-in-law's support. But I missed my own mother, and I wished that she had been there to mother me, as I took my first steps into motherhood.

There is the chance that you could make those lost futures into something else, altogether. Jennifer recently told me that her whole family were going on a trip to Madeira. Her father had always wanted to go there but had died before making the dream a reality - so this became a kind of pilgrimage for them.

You may also find that relationships with your brothers and sisters will change. Old conflicts may resurface, or dissolve. Parents often act as reporters from one member of the family to another. Without that flow of information it becomes your choice to maintain the relationship for yourself – or not. This is an opportunity and can be a good thing. I am less lazy about communicating with my brother and sisters than I would have been if Mum were still sending out a newsletter on what everyone was up to. I feel that we have become closer as a result, and I hope they feel the same.

Wills can also be a huge source of argument. Of course your parents' money and assets are theirs to do with exactly as they wished. Even so, if there are rivalries or bitterness between the children, it seems that this is where they will come out. Many of Agatha Christie's best mysteries were based on rivalries surrounding an inheritance! Those who look for it can always find unfairness, and sometimes people do behave atrociously, too.

A death in the family will not change people's personalities, and may make worse any faults. Everyone's emotions are raw at this time. My only thoughts here are that none of us is 'entitled' to an inheritance. You will, however, want to make sure that your parents' wishes are honoured if you can. If you disagree with their choices of how to leave their money, please forgive them. Your own sanity is precious beyond price. If you have a disagreement with other family members, only you can know when it is best to let go and concentrate on your life now.

Losing a Sibling or Friend

On the surface the loss of a sibling or friend may seem a 'lesser' trauma than the death of a partner or a parent. However, it depends on your relationship, and there are other factors involved here. It has often been said that we can choose our friends, but not our family. So the loss of a friend involves the disappearance of someone you spent time with because you wanted to. You may have spent the time of your friend's illness feeling at a loss as to how to help, and wished you had been able to do more. You may also be involved with supporting other loved ones – a partner or child who has been bereaved for instance.

It may seem difficult to address your own grief, as you busy yourself caring for others. In this case, check to see that you are taking care of your own needs – which are just as valid as those of the people that society may regard as 'closer' to the deceased. Look over the stages of grief and tasks of mourning described above. Some or all of these will apply to you too. By all means offer your support to others, as long as you are looking after yourself and your own mourning too.

It may also be that your friend was part of your support network. If so you will have to take a look at that. You may find you now become closer to other friends, or to family. You may have to rely more on your own ingenuity. If you can stay open, caring and giving, you will be able to build new supports for the future.

Losing a sibling changes the energy in your family. If this is the first of your generation to die, it may seem a death knell for you all. Who will be next? If you are the only remaining sibling, you may feel you are now on borrowed time. Confronting our own mortality can be scary, if we let it. Or it can be liberating.

A colleague, John, once asked for my advice and support when his sister was dying of cancer, knowing about my history with my mother. This lady was only in her early forties. John's sharing of his experience gave me food for thought. It left me with the phrase "Life is just too short – at least try to find what you want" drifting through my mind. What I wanted was a relationship with a wonderful man - to whom I have now been married for eleven years. That experience of staring reality (even though someone else's) in the face changed my whole life!

If you have lost a brother or sister, you may find that there are unresolved conflicts still in your family. Immediately after someone dies, emotions may be running high. It would be wise to give everyone the benefit of the doubt at this time, and let the dust settle a little. You do have an opportunity to reach out to other family members.

Remember that being loved is one of our most sought after

experiences as human beings, and that we gain love best by giving it away.

Losing a Child

The death of your child is a pain beyond describing. Any parent can feel the wrenching of their heart when they even consider such a possibility. Even when the child is an adult, there is a sense that their death is outside the natural progression. You experience immense resistance. It isn't *supposed* to happen that way. No one expects to have to deal with the emotions surrounding the death of their child. We are totally unprepared.

If you have lost your child when they are not yet adult, there is an extra difficulty in letting them go. It is hard for you to imagine them other than as you last saw them. They appear to be frozen in time – development stopped at the age at which they died.

Always your baby

If you believe in life after death you may worry what will happen to them. Are they stuck forever as a child? It may be helpful to picture them continuing to grow and age in the spirit world. They will live out their lives there, and grow into young adults. However they will never experience some of the challenges of life, and so will remain more innocent and childlike in their outlook. This may be a comfort to you, and it may be helpful to keep track as the birthdays pass. If you find it difficult to picture them as they grow, photos of yourself or their other parent at the same age may help. Though your child is not a carbon copy of you, they may have something of your looks.

It is most important to focus on what you did experience

together, rather than on the events you will not now share. I once worked with Manuel, whose child was diagnosed with severe spina bifida whilst in the womb. He and his wife chose to carry the baby to term, knowing their little one would die within days of birth. They knew they were giving their child the gift of that time with them, along with their love in the short months of pregnancy, and in the days before he died. It was a wonderful gift for their son, and having him in their lives was a gift for them. They will always have that to remember.

Losing a child will never be easy, as the bond runs so deep. It will help if you share your feelings, especially with the other parent and any other children. Above all let those who are still here know that you love them as well. They can still benefit from knowing how much you care.

Society's Attitude

Reactions to death vary from culture to culture. Some mourn loudly; others batten down the hatches on their emotions. Some celebrate the life of the deceased with a wake or party; others mourn the loss of a shared future. Some cultural approaches to death seem to be more helpful than others. The good news is that we can learn from the best of other cultures.

In the West we tend to sweep emotions under the carpet, rather than expressing them. We can learn from cultures where it is seen as acceptable to let those emotions out rather than suppressing them. As a society, we also tend to regard death as a tragedy. We can also learn from cultures where death is seen as natural, or even a joy for those passing on. We can learn to celebrate our loved one's life.

In our society today there seems to be a 'statute of limitations' on grieving. It is understood that you will find life challenging in the days and weeks after the death of a loved one, but not that you may become suddenly grief-stricken a year later and find it impossible to get out of bed for a week.

The only cure for this attitude of others is to let them have their attitude, but don't judge yourself by it. Grieving takes how long it takes. You can choose to move through it by dealing with your own emotions, but this is a time to be kind to yourself. Queen Victoria continued to wear black in mourning for her beloved Prince Albert for forty years until her own death. Nobody but you can say when you are ready to move forward with your life, though I hope it will be before forty years have passed.

Separating Current from Past Grief

One aspect of grief that may come as a surprise is its ability to rekindle old hurts. Loss of a partner may trigger renewed grief over losing a parent, or vice versa. This will happen most when you have not processed your feelings fully during the earlier loss.

This can also happen even if the loss you suffered before was not a death. Unresolved issues from a divorce, moving homes or traumas from childhood may all resurface. These feelings are reappearing because they feel related, and are still somehow stored inside you. "Oh good," says your subconscious. "You're handling all this grief, can you deal with this left over bit too?"

It is important here to recognise the complication for what it is. Your job is to see that unfinished business from your past is affecting how you feel now. You can identify the feelings that relate to past issues and deal with them, just as you have learned to handle your feelings in this book. See Chapter 6 for further details. Once you have taken steps to identify and move through or let go of feelings from your past, you will then be better able to continue through the stages of this current grief.

Constant Reminders

Undoubtedly the hardest times when you are mourning someone dear to you are the ones when you are directly reminded of that person. Even making tea or coffee can be painful, when you fetch only one cup from the cupboard. Whoever the person was to you, there will always be times, places, words and smells that remind you especially of them.

In the early days of bereavement, life will seem like a series of 'unfulfilled moments'. You are about to pick up the phone to call your mother, then realise she is no longer there to call. You find you have made two cups of coffee without even thinking about it. You can't quite bring yourself to do anything particular on a Thursday evening, because that's when you always played cards with Bob.

Perhaps you think that the best approach is to avoid as many reminders as possible. There may be ways to do this, see **Creating New Patterns** below. It would be wise, however, to avoid throwing out everything that reminds you of them straight away. By all means put their things to one side, so you don't have to keep mentally tripping over them. But don't be in too much of a hurry to go through them. With a little time and perspective, some of those things can help you to create precious memories.

As time goes by, and sooner if you choose, those reminders can become times to recall your loved one. You can dwell on the good times you shared, and what you meant to each other. You get to edit your thoughts, and can make the effort to linger on the pleasant memories. So when you feel the pain of an unfulfilled moment, for now just reassure yourself that there will be a time when you will be glad to think of your loved one.

Letting Them Go

Either you believe in the continuation of our spirit after death or you don't. I'm not aiming to change your beliefs either way. So if you are a die-hard 'no such thing as life after death' person, it's probably better to skip onto the next section. However, if you are unsure, or convinced that life does go on in some way, there is something to consider. I have already covered the fact that your grief is mainly about you, not the person who has died (see **Accept That They Are OK** above). This is true, and the main reason to process your emotions is so that you can move through the stages of grief and build your new life.

I personally believe that our spirit does continue after death. For me it just seems impossible to accept that my body alone is what makes me 'Me'. My spirit seems much stronger than this (however wonderful) contraption of flesh and bones that moves me around.

Assuming that spirit continues after death, what will the spirit of your departed be doing now? Chances are that they will be trying to comfort you, as I described earlier. I believe their job is to move on to their new life, the same as yours. And yet, this could be very hard for them if you are struggling with your grief. Can you see anything of yourself here? Are you holding back the spirit of your loved one because it is hard for you to let them go? Wanting the best for them can give you an incentive to move through your grief, so they can heal too.

This doesn't mean there is anything wrong with talking to them, but it should be done with the intention of finishing business and letting go. After all, this is the reason we hold a funeral. The ritual of saying goodbye is a comfort and can be useful in providing an ending.

You have to say goodbye in your heart as well.

Creating New Patterns

I want you to nurture yourself! Some of the new patterns you make in your life must be devoted to you – to taking care of your needs. Whether those needs are for counselling or for chocolate cake (or both!), it is up to you to attend to them.

Now your old life is changed beyond recognition, there is an opportunity to throw out the rule book. In my experience, very few people are self-indulgent. We tend to put others first. For many of us it is a real challenge to do anything for ourselves. If we do, we often feel guilty. This is a good time to do something about that.

You have been bereaved. You need looking after.

It would be nice if you had others running round after you, but the truth is that others are also bereaved, and have their own agenda. Alternatively, there just may not be anyone there to comfort you. So how can you look after your own needs?

This is also a time to look at the rituals in your life. Which of them support you, and which are of no help? You will probably find there are many things that you do in a certain way out of habit. Perhaps they are not working to support you. Some may even be done that way because of the person who has died. Now is your opportunity to change. There is no need to keep doing things in someone else's way as some kind of a punishment.

As you move into the recovery stage of your grief, it is time to try some new activities. Maybe you could join a group you have been meaning to try. One word of caution, though. However passionate you are about a cause, I would avoid spending too much time on activities related to cancer, at least in the early days. Supporting your local hospice or volunteering to fundraise for a cancer charity may be great further down the line. In the early days, though, it will keep you stuck in a mindset of pain. It's not nurturing you at this stage. It would be better to focus on positive activities – even rekindle a long lost interest or hobby if you haven't done so already.

As in everything, balance is key. You will want to keep some old routines in your life. There is a need for some stability. Keep some familiar activities, as they will make you feel more secure.

As I mentioned before, you may also be learning to handle jobs that were once the responsibility of the person who has died. Remember that you may be able to 'outsource' some of these. There is no reason why you should have to mow your own lawn, if you can afford to pay someone to do it for you. What do you now have on your plate that someone could help you with? When you do take on new activities, remember to give yourself credit. Build your confidence in your abilities. Start with little things. Congratulate yourself for remembering to lock up at night, and you will gain confidence to tackle the 'larger' things as you go along.

Finding Strength Within

The disappearance of someone you love from your life is a testing time. It may feel as though you have been abandoned – possibly even by God, or whatever you think of as a Universal Power. Many people have wondered how a loving God could visit tragedies upon them. Many others have found instead a source of faith and comfort. At this time it can help to turn to your faith, or be open to finding one. If you can trust that life is unfolding as it should, if you can bear what has been put before you, you will give yourself time to adjust.

We all have an inner reserve, whether we believe this comes from ourselves, or somewhere 'out there'. You can tap into this strength if you let yourself. Trust that the strength you need will come – maybe not now, but in time. If you do not feel able to cope, as I suggested earlier on try 'borrowing' the strength of someone you admire. How did Nelson Mandela cope with imprisonment and degradation for all those years, for instance? What inner reserves allowed him to continue to believe in the good in people? By reading what someone has written, even by speaking their words, you can put yourself into their mindset, and take on some of their strengths.

Living Your Own Life from Now On

Everyone is living his or her own life. And yet often you may find that you put someone else at the centre of your thoughts. This can happen especially when someone is ill. Your loved one has probably been much in your mind. Your life may even have begun to revolve around their needs. So what now? Now, you have to begin living for yourself. This doesn't mean you stop caring for others. It doesn't mean you can't help others who are also bereaved. It means that you take responsibility for your life and happiness. It means that you can do things your loved one would not like or approve of, if they are right for you.

Some fall into the temptation to begin living life, in some way, for the person who has died. I met Miriam, from New York, at a seminar in Los Angeles, and over lunch we compared life stories. I discovered that her mother had died of cancer at much the same age as mine. As I described to Miriam my journey to believing that death was fine for my mother, she looked surprised. I told her that I felt that for Mum it was fine for her life to end then.

Then the light went on for Miriam. She was a nutritionist, and she was trying to save *everybody* from her mother's fate. Now, maybe being a nutritionist was what she really wanted to do with her life, and maybe she would continue. But Miriam realised that she had in some way been living her life for someone else. She was still trying to fix her Mum.

So whilst it is great to use your experience to create meaning in your life, it has to be your purpose. It can only truly be *your* purpose if you are able to let the person go, as I have described above.

Continuing Support Strategies

By now you should have a full support team. You may have been keeping a journal, enlisting the help of friends, have a life coach or use complementary therapies. Whatever it is that works for you. It is important to continue with these supports for as long as you need them. This could be months, years, or the rest of your life!

This may also be the time to add in extra supports. Possibly in the past you were able to 'just get on with it', but now feel that your world is falling apart. This may be the time to add counselling to your support structure, or some of the other methods detailed in Chapter 6.

If you want to take control of your progress through grief, it may help to hire a life coach to support you. Coaching does not have to be all about action - but it will help you to look at the life you would like to build, get back in touch with your own needs, and take the first steps when you are ready.

Grief is very hidden in Western society. People will probably assume that after a few months you are 'over' your loss. They won't know that you need someone to listen years later as you express emotions that are still surfacing then. You could let friends or family know when you are having a tough time. They may just need you to ask in order to offer the support you need.

There is no time limit on grief, or on the need for counselling. As I mentioned earlier emotions can resurface many years after a traumatic event, especially when triggered by another difficult time in your life. It is never too late to let the emotion flow so you can process it, let it go and move on.

Keep Them in Your Heart

This is the last of William Worden's tasks of mourning, and the most pleasant. He describes it as 'emotionally relocating the deceased'. I like to think of it as making a place for them in your heart. Choosing to remember the good parts of your relationship. Keeping the best and letting go of the rest. You can create positive memories. Not with the purpose of making yourself feel worse about your loss, but in order to feel the joy of having had that person in your life.

I would like to give the last words of this chapter to somebody else. When I began writing this book, I found the words of this song inspirational. It would be equally appropriate when your loved one is dying, or when they are already gone. It is a beautiful song, written by Julie Blue for the eight-month-old son of a friend, when he was dying.

I hope the words touch you too, and suggest you do what you can to hear them sung by Julie herself (you can buy her CD of the same title):

A Wing And A Prayer (for Camilo)

I'm thinking of you, I see your face so clearly
I've got you in my heart, I hold you dearly
I'm surrounding you with so much light
You can't help but know that I care
I'm sending you – a wing and a prayer

Coming through the darkness

Shining like a star

Coming to remember

Who you really are

Beyond this life you are a spirit

Who never dies so do not fear it

Or the truth when you hear it

I'm thinking of you, I see your face so clearly

I've got you in my heart, I hold you dearly

I'm surrounding you with so much light

You can't help but know that I care

I'm sending you – a wing and a prayer

Wing and a prayer, a wing and a prayer

I'm trying to get quiet

Trying to be still

Searching for the silence

So I can listen until

I hear a voice inside me

Whisper tender words to guide me

Knowing you'll always be beside me

I'm thinking of you

I'm thinking of all the lives you touched

And how much poorer we'd all be

Without having known you

We're thinking of you

We see your face so clearly

We've got you in our hearts

We hold you dearly

We're surrounding you with so much love

You can't help but know that we care

We're sending you – a wing and a prayer

Wing and a prayer, a wing and a prayer

ACTION STEP

Create a memorial to your departed one. This could be a photo album, a poem, a picture, or a letter about what they meant to you. Keep this memorial to help you make that space in your heart for the person you loved.

10

A TIME OF REFLECTION AND REBUILDING

Arriving at your destination – wherever it may be – is the end of the journey itself, but it's not the end of your life. Now you've arrived, you move into a time of consolidation: time to reflect on what's gone before, and to get to know this new place in which you're going to spend the next part of your life.

Time for Grounding in Your New Scenery

I've already compared your journey to fleeing a natural disaster, which makes me realise that this arrival is not so different from moving house (though almost certainly more emotional). When you move to a new area, you have to get used to a totally new environment. You have left behind all that is comfortable. Nothing is as familiar as it was in your old home.

Even simple tasks such as having your hair cut can involve research or risk as you try out something new. You are thrown back on your own resources, as you don't have a support network built up in this new place. Everything starts off unfamiliar and strange, but as time goes by you find new resources and make new connections. You regain a sense of control and choice as you explore your new area. You can speed up the process by having the courage to go out and take the risk of trying new experiences. You can be open to help, support and friendship from others. You can also connect more quickly with your new landscape by spending time there – by walking and really looking at what is here in this new space, with curiosity and openness.

In the same way, you now need to ground yourself in the scenery that appears at the destination of your journey with your loved one's cancer. What parts of life are similar to when you set off, and what has changed? As you go through this grounding process, it will also reinforce many of the important parts of the journey itself.

Reflect on What You Learned

Taking the Inner Journey is a brave thing to do. Most people you will meet in your day-to-day life will not have done this. They are either numb to their feelings, or at their mercy. They may feel a yearning for something that is missing from their lives, or even suffer in various ways with their health as a result.

You have taken that journey, and along the way you are sure

to have learned many things. So now take some time to reflect. Look back on where you were before the journey began. This will make the lessons you have learned clear to you now. One of the many things you may have learned is what *matters* to you in your life. You could also know a lot more about your true capabilities. Imagine tapping into the reserves you have found whenever you need to, as you go forward in your life.

You have probably also discovered much about your relationships with people around you. These relationships will have been revealed to be strong or weak, and hopefully you will already have found ways to make them deeper and stronger.

Living the Lessons

The only way to make the lessons you have learned meaningful is to live them out in your life as you go forward. Otherwise they will be like all the school books you may have gathering dust in your attic – no use to anyone. When was the last time you applied what you learned in school maths? Does there seem any point now in knowing how to calculate the length of the hypotenuse? Was it worth the time you spent getting that education? Well, it may have been, if it taught you *how to learn*. This is one of the greatest life skills you can have. My husband often reminds me that what counts is not what you know – it's what you know how to find out. Your Inner Journey has taught you how to learn emotionally.

Whatever you haven't learned already, you can spend the rest of your life learning. Most deep thinkers will tell you that they regard learning as a life-long process. Albert Einstein said, "The more I learn, the more I realise I don't know".

Just keep in mind that there is no point in learning any of it unless it makes a difference in your life. Then it will also make a difference for the people around you. It's no good knowing that relationships are based on open communication (for example) and then keeping that insight to yourself, is it?

Keep applying what you have learned as you move forwards. Above all use it to work on the areas you have realised are most important to you. For the majority of people that will be the relationships they build with those around them. Your relationships may need attention. It may be that during your journey you paid more attention to some relationships than others. Perhaps your family came first and you didn't have as much time for your friends. If there are any people you've been neglecting, now is the time to use your improved communication skills to deal with that.

It would also be good to continue your inner journey. This journey never ends until you arrive at your essential core, and feel a sense of profound peace at all times. This is something that few have achieved in our world so far, and yet I feel that we live at a time where more and more people are taking this journey. We are becoming closer and more connected to our spiritual natures.

This is ultimately the way to heal us all, and heal the world into the bargain.

Skills You Have Gained

Along with the lessons you have learned, you will also have practised some amazing new skills. This can be hard for you to appreciate if you feel critical of what you achieved during your journey with your loved one's cancer. Instead of focusing on what you didn't do, or what you got wrong, try looking at what you got right. Acknowledge the times when you were patient beyond belief, and the determination you showed in taking on more tasks when you wanted to be doing something else.

Notice how your communication skills have improved. Congratulate yourself for every time you heard what someone was really saying underneath the words they spoke. Having empathy with another human being is a skill that you shouldn't underestimate. If you kept on going whatever happened, or stayed calm in the face of stress and troubles, these are also wonderful skills.

Some supporters find that if they have been caring for a loved one full time, they face a challenge in getting back into work when that role is over. I can't prevent that being true – or overturn the prejudice you might find as a result of a 'gap' in your CV. The most important factor, though, is that *you* value what you have done. Rather than leaving a gap, put on your CV some of the skills you have gained.

This is much like it is for a mother going back to work after time at home raising small children. She has to have confidence in herself, first, before her prospective employers can do so. For many mothers in this situation, the decision they take is to keep their earning power in their own hands. They take control by starting their own businesses. This may seem like an enormous stretch for you now, but there has never been a time when there was more opportunity to earn money from home. If you want to take this approach, find out what resources are available to you locally and learn, learn, learn.

Of course, there's more to life than work and business.

Perhaps your new direction will include travel, voluntary work at home or overseas or pursuing a passion – now that you know what is important to you.

Your Life is Precious

One of the main reasons I wrote this book was that as I researched books on cancer, I discovered we were largely missing - those of us who haven't battled the disease ourselves may be mentioned, but always after the person who has cancer. I wanted to correct the balance.

Of course the cancer host is important – they are dear to you, or you wouldn't care what happened to them. You are equally important. The world wouldn't be the same without you in it. Have you ever seen the film *It's A Wonderful Life* with James Stewart? It's one of our favourites. The main character (who is contemplating suicide) is given an opportunity by his guardian angel. He gets the chance to see what other people's lives would be like without him in the world. As he sees the way the smallest actions he made rippled out to affect the lives of others, his faith in the meaning of his own life is restored. Your life is just as important as his.

I hope you have been taking notice of the message in this book that *you* are important, and have been taking good care of yourself. Whatever the outcome of your loved one's cancer, you are still of value. If they have recovered and don't seem to need you as much, don't feel let down. Now you get to share life and future times together as equals. If they are gone, well *you* are not. You will have much to give to the world in the future, when you are ready. You create the meaning in your life, and that life is precious.

Everything is Unfolding as it Should

One night I was driving home after an evening out, and the Beatles song *All You Need Is Love* came on the radio. Now in my teens I loved The Beatles. I knew all the words to the songs and would sing along, but I hadn't listened to this song for a very long time. The words really struck me. In between the repetitions of the simple chorus are some deep thoughts, and the one that springs to my mind now is the line "There's nowhere you can be that isn't where you were meant to be".

So wherever your destination may be, you were meant to be here. Once you accept this as true, there is no longer any need to resist. You didn't choose this challenge, but it was the way your life turned out. It doesn't mean you wanted it that way, but here it is. Being at peace with that makes it easy, as The Beatles say.

If you are still resisting the situation, try writing down some of the things you think should be a different way. One possibility could be "My loved one should still be here with me". If they are not, you can't change that reality. Resisting it is pointless, and just makes you feel worse. See if you can reframe the things you have written – turn them around to read a different way. For instance "I accept that my loved one is no longer here and I choose to keep happy memories of them." You can also use any methods that have helped you in your Inner Journey to continue dissolving your resistance.

Let Go of Regret

In addition to resisting the current situation, we often spend a lot of energy resisting the past. As if it could make any difference! It is a waste of that energy to deny the reality of the past. Regret over what has happened is one way that we resist. If you spend time wishing that things had been different – that your loved one had had more fight, or hadn't risked their health by some behaviour in the past, all you are doing is holding yourself back. Don't regret this journey you have made; it will help you if you can try to find the positive in it. Resisting will slow up your adjustment to your new scenery.

Take the example of my friend Angelina. She had to move because of her husband's job, at around the same time I was moving to be by the sea. In her case, the town she was moving to would not be on your list of top ten destinations in the UK. She could have regretted the move or been jealous of me, but all that would have done was to give her a bad attitude to her new home. Who would have wanted to get to know her then? Why would anyone befriend someone who plainly doesn't want to be there?

Instead she made the best of things. She accepted the benefits of her husband's better job. She no longer had to go out to work, and could be home to collect her children from school. Not such a bad thing at all. Letting go of that regret allowed her to adjust more quickly to her new scenery. You can do the same.

Delight in Your Life

As you move forward in your life from this point you know

something that many others don't. At least, they do know it, but mostly choose to ignore it. You have realised that life is short. Too short to be spent fighting, putting things off or mistreating anyone, least of all people you care about.

Make your life have meaning by appreciating the people around you, and relishing every moment. Life could be taken away at any time, so savour what you have now.

Keep Connected to Nature

In Chapter 5 I talked about the benefits of being connected to nature. It calms you and gives you a sense of your own place in nature. The native Americans have long known this. Chief Luther Standing Bear said, "The old Lakota was wise. He knew that man's heart away from nature becomes hard; he knew that lack of respect for growing, living things soon led to lack of respect for humans, too. So he kept his children close to nature's softening influence."

As you continue onwards, keep this influence in *your* life, too. There is always a way to do this. A single stone is as much a part of nature as the highest mountain. You can get miniature Zen gardens or indoor fountains, which will fit into the tiniest of spaces. There are parks in every city. Taking time to walk from one place to another will not only keep you fit but also allow you the time to notice the natural environment around you. I love to look at the raindrops on a shiny leaf, or the crashing waves - so you don't even need good weather.

Many of the same benefits can be gained from art (yours or other people's), calming or uplifting music or your connection to your spiritual nature.

Looking After Yourself

As I have already said, your life is precious. You play a valuable and unique part in our world. So it is important that you look after yourself. It's not necessary for you to go on the same journey as your loved one. You have made your own journey and that is as it should be.

As you move forward into your new life, continue to respect the body in which you find yourself. Look after your physical health. In the early days this may mean plenty of rest, then increasing levels of exercise in line with your improving strength. Maintain the good nutrition patterns you have started. My father kept up with the diet he and my mother adopted when she was ill, and it has improved his health greatly in the long term. In fact he is pleased to have now outlived the age his own father reached.

Looking after yourself doesn't only revolve around your body. Your mind and spirit need nourishment as well. Listen to yourself to find what your other needs are, and then find creative and fun ways to fill those needs.

Focus on What You *Do* Want

Because what you focus on expands, it is vital to make sure that you are concentrating on things that you want to happen, rather than on your fears. Whilst accepting the parts of your life that are outside your control, you can choose to look at what you would like to happen. After all, you can't focus on what you want if you don't know what that is.

Revisit the Wheel of Life chart shown in Chapter 4 regularly. Give your life a score in each of the areas. Then imagine what it would be like if you were to count a ten in that area. What would your career or your relationship be like then?

The most important thing is to look at possibilities. Even if your score of ten in that area is not possible right now, what is the easiest way you can attain the essential elements of your vision in the shortest time?

Sharing Your Insights

One way to add meaning to your life as you go forward is to share what you have learned with others. This can be directly by talking to people who are open to what you learned. Or it can be simply by example - in the way you live your life.

This journey you have made will not be in vain if you use it to create ripples out into the world. What ripples will you make? (You are always making ripples whether you care to or not!) Will they be ripples of negativity, distrust and fear – or ripples of acceptance, peace and calm? You get to choose, but I hope you will go for the second choice, because I'm likely to be on the receiving end of some of those ripples.

If you feel you still have some negative emotions, and you now know better than to suppress them, continue to work on your Inner Journey for as long as it takes. If you have to complain, use your Hard Times Notebook (see Chapter 6), and don't transfer those negative vibes to anyone else.

Make sure that the insights you share are for the greater good of others, not to tell them what to do and add levels of duty to their lives.

Be Responsible for Your Own Happiness

Many teachers, such as His Holiness the Dalai Lama, Lester Levenson and author Robert Holden, have told us that happiness is not a product of events outside us. It comes from within – from our own interpretation of the events in our lives. It's your job (not anyone else's) to make your own happiness.

You will find that if you're happy, everything around you seems to mysteriously improve, especially your relationships - everyone loves to be around happy people. If you are struggling with the idea that you could be happy, remember that not everything in your life has to be perfect for you to be happy in one particular moment. If you can leave the past and future alone just for now and focus on the present, you can be happy.

Try eating an ice cream in the sunshine. Concentrate on nothing but the sensations that brings (or even watch a child who is doing this – they certainly know how to be happy). Have a laugh with a friend. Take a long candlelit bath. Do anything that makes you conscious of *now*, rather than regrets about the past or fears of the future.

We have been taught to believe that our happiness depends on perfect situations or the way others behave, but that kind of thinking is a Catch-22. Often by being happy we would improve those outside conditions. Happiness in the moment even improves health, as I described when I talked about humour in Chapter 5.

I used an exercise in one of my workshops that covers this aspect of happiness:

- First you write down what you are making your happiness depend on — for instance "I would be happy if I weighed twenty pounds less".

- Then you turn it around to say "If I were happy, I would be more likely to exercise, and then I would reach my ideal body weight".

Try a more challenging example. "I would be happy if my partner (or mother, brother, son etc.) were still alive." You can't have the thing you crave, so you are ensuring that you will never be happy. It is still possible to turn this around, for example, "If I were happy, I would make more friends, and cope better without my partner."

Once you have turned things around like this it is very freeing — because you no longer have to sort everything out! Instead you can relax, and focus on finding activities that you feel happy doing. My wish is that you create a happy future — starting **NOW**.

ACTION STEP

Look back through your journal, or at anything you drew or wrote during your journey. Reflect on how far you have come and how you have grown, then visualise the path ahead.

Bring that new you into today by doing something that you really enjoy. Remember to notice how happy you feel while you are doing it.

11

T.I.I.S.G. – PASSING IT ON

T.I.I.S.G. What on earth does that mean? I first came across this expression in Joe Vitale's book *The Attractor Factor*. He explained that it stands for Turn It Into Something Good. The best way to put meaning into something challenging that happens in your life is to Turn It Into Something Good.

There are those who think that some events are just too awful to ever produce something good, but they are wrong. Just as manure can produce the most beautiful roses, so the worst events that happen in our lives can act as fertiliser for greater things to come.

I have already shared one example of this transformation with you, the example of Immaculée Ilibagiza in Chapter 7. She has transformed her terrible experiences in the Rwandan genocide in order to teach compassion and forgiveness to others.

Diana Lamplugh is another example. She is the mother of Suzy Lamplugh, who was an estate agent from Birmingham in the UK. Someone posing as a client abducted Suzy and, it is presumed, killed her. Diana and her husband Paul used this incredibly painful experience. They set up the Suzy Lamplugh Trust, which now advises on safety for everyone. It has undoubtedly saved many lives since.

One of the most famous examples of recent times has been the 'Calendar Girls' of Yorkshire. Their story has been made into a fabulous film, so you may already know it, but I'll tell the story again here in brief.

The Calendar Girls' Story

Up until 1998 Angela Baker and Tricia Stewart were just normal Yorkshire women. Tricia worked with her husband in their own business, and both women attended their local Women's Institute meetings.

Everything changed when Angela's husband John was diagnosed with non-Hodgkins lymphoma (a blood-related cancer). During his illness, Tricia joked with John that they should produce an alternative WI calendar to raise funds for the hospital, with the ladies posing in the nude. John thought it was a cracking idea, a celebration of the beauty of the women of Yorkshire, but he never believed they would do it.

After John's death, the idea resurfaced, and eleven brave ladies went ahead with creating the calendar. These ladies took their clothes off in spite of their fears of the disapproval of the Women's

Institute. The massive publicity they generated meant that the calendar went on to sell hundreds of thousands of copies in the UK and the USA. Many others have also imitated the idea since then. A film production revitalised interest years later and another calendar was produced. So far, the Calendar Girls have raised nearly £2 million for Leukaemia Research. You can read more about how these 'ordinary women' produced such extraordinary results in Tricia Stewart's book *Calendar Girl*.

What About the Small Stuff?

All these examples may seem to you to be on a very large scale. You may be tempted to think that 'little old me' could never achieve anything like that. If so, I'm sure that you are wrong.

None of these people seemed destined for greatness. The only difference between them and others (for whom challenge has appeared but hasn't yet been turned into something good) is that they took some action – based on inspiration.

It is important, though, to remember the small stuff too. Turning it into something good could be as simple as an extra hug for your children when they leave your house, or spending more time with a friend. Even attending to your own happiness, as I recommended in Chapter 10, is turning it into something good.

Lester Levenson (the creator of the Sedona Method, whom we first met in Chapter 5) said, "One person with only love in his or her heart could do more to right the problems of the world than all the people who are actively trying to fix it." If you have love in your heart you stop being part of the problem, so you automatically become part of the solution.

Now it's Over to You

How do you go about it? What are the steps you need to take to Turn It Into Something Good? I'm sure there are as many methods or procedures as there are people, but I can share with you how it happened for me. (Yes, I consider this book - and the creation of Families Facing Cancer - to be my T.I.I.S.G.)

Here are the steps of the process.

1. *Set your intention.*

    Once you decide that you want to T.I.I.S.G., this will set your subconscious mind onto the task. Your 'autopilot' will look tirelessly for ways for you to do this, without you needing to give any concentration to it whatsoever. I think that this step is the one I rather missed out on, because I wasn't aware I wanted to be using this process. Perhaps that is why I am doing this so many years after my mother died. I am convinced that taking this step will shorten the process for you.

2. *Get on with your life, while you wait for inspiration.*

    As you already know, I spent many years after my mother died just getting on with my life. Fifteen years of living, loving, learning, growing and later trying to live up to my son's view of me as 'the best Mum in the world'.

    It's no good pushing for inspiration. Don't worry about it. This is the time when you can focus on the small stuff, which is in fact the biggest of all, and live the best life you can; build the best relationships you can; do what you can to be happy. All of this is important too.

3. *When inspiration arrives, take some action.*

    This doesn't mean you have to plunge out of your comfort zone straight away – but only by taking the first step will you ever find out what destination you are aiming for, let alone how to get there. My inspiration arrived in 2006, and it was totally unexpected. I first thought of writing a book around the subject of cancer when I applied for a job as a fundraiser at my local hospice. The hospice director gave the job to someone better qualified, but the book idea stayed and took root. In my case the first step was research. I started reading books on the subject of cancer, to see what I would be able to add. It wasn't until a year later that the second inspiration hit – the knowledge of who I was writing the book for. I would never have had that second inspiration if I hadn't been prepared to take the first steps.

4. *Find a system to continue the action.*

    Having found the certainty inside me of what I wanted to create, I began to take one step after another. It wasn't until I found the system that worked for me, however, that things really began to take off. In my case this came from reading and implementing the book *Wishcraft* by Barbara Sher, which I have referred to already. You could also use the exercises in her book to shorten the inspiration process, as they guide you towards realising what you want to achieve.

    If you already have a system for achieving your goals, then use that. If you have an inspiration to go for a goal that seems big and scary, then you could hire a life coach to help and support you in reaching it. Personally I think big goals are in some ways easier than small ones. Big goals are worth putting in an effort for; other people care about them too, which means you get more help; and they seem somehow to develop a momentum of their own.

5. *Spread the word*

    When you know what your T.I.I.S.G. is (be it big and breathtaking, or small and sweet), and you're taking action towards it, don't keep it to yourself. Write and let me know about it. Post it on our forums and generally tell the world. You may even get some help in making it happen. Joe Vitale told me to T.I.I.S.G, and I've passed it on from me to you. Now it's your turn to pass it on to whoever comes next.

Recommended Reading

Bach, Richard. *Illusions: The Adventures of a Reluctant Messiah.* Arrow
Books Ltd, 2001.

Byrne, Rhonda. *The Secret.* Simon & Schuster Ltd, 2006.

Chopra, Deepak. *Quantum Healing: Exploring the Frontiers of Mind/Body
Spirit.* Bantam Books, 1989.

Chopra, Deepak. *The Book Of Secrets.* Rider & Co, 2004.

Coelho, Paulo. *The Alchemist.* Harper Collins, Australia, 1993.

Cooke, Helen (Rev.) *The Bristol Approach To Living With Cancer.*
Robinson Publishing, 2003.

Covey, Stephen. *The 8th Habit: From Effectiveness to Greatness.* Simon &
Schuster Ltd, 2004.

Cutler, Howard and His Holiness The Dalai Lama. *The Art Of
Happiness: A Handbook For Living.* Hodder & Stoughton Ltd,
1998

Dwoskin, Hale and Levenson, Lester. *Happiness Is Free, and It's Easier
Than You Think!* Sedona Press, 2002.

Dwoskin, Hale. *The Sedona Method: Your Key to Lasting Happiness, Success,
Peace and Emotional Well-being.* Sedona Press, 2003.

Frankl, Viktor. *Man's Search For Meaning.* Beacon Press, 1993.

Grason, Sandy. *Journalution: Journal Writing to Heal Your Life and Manifest Your Dreams.* New World Library, 2005.

Hall, Alvin. *Money For Life: Everyone's Guide to Financial Freedom.* Coronet Books, 2000.

Holden, Robert. *Happiness Now!: Timeless Wisdom For Feeling Good Fast.* Hodder & Stoughton Ltd, 1998.

Hutton, Deborah. *What Can I Do To Help? : 75 Practical Ideas for Family and Friends from Cancer's Frontline.* Short Books, 2005.

Ilibagiza, Immaculée. *Left To Tell: Discovering God Amidst the Rwandan Holocaust.* Hay House, 2006.

Jenkinson, Audrey. *Past Caring.* Polperro Heritage Press, 2004.

Katie, Byron. *Loving What Is: Four Questions That Can Change Your Life.* Harmony, 2002.

Macbeth, Jessica Williams. *Moon Over Water : Meditation Made Clear With Techniques For Beginners And Initiates.* Gateway, 1990.

Marriott, Hugh. *The Selfish Pig's Guide To Caring.* Time Warner Paperbacks, 2006.

McKay, Judith and Hirano, Nancee. *The Chemotherapy and Radiation Therapy Survival Guide.* New Harbinger Publications, 1993.

Sher, Barbara and Gottlieb, Annie. *Wishcraft : How To Get What You Really Want.* Viking Press, 1979.

Simpson, Joe. *Touching The Void.* Jonathan Cape Ltd, 1988.

Stewart, Tricia. *Calendar Girl.* Sidgwick & Jackson Ltd, 2001.

Virtue, Doreen. *Constant Craving: What Your Food Cravings Mean and How to Overcome Them.* Hay House Inc, 1995.

Vitale, Joe. *The Attractor Factor: 5 Easy Steps for Creating Wealth (or Anything Else) from the Inside Out.* John Wiley & Sons, 2005.

Wilson, Paul. *Calm For Life.* Penguin Books Ltd, 2000.

Wishart, Adam. *One In Three: A Son's Journey into the Science and History of Cancer.* Profile Books Ltd, 2006.

Index

About The Author

Anne Orchard is a life coach based in Dorset, UK, whose areas of expertise include offering support to those affected by illness or death of a loved one and helping them to rebuild their lives. Following the death of her mother from cancer in 1991, and her mother-in-law's experience of breast cancer in 2004, Anne became increasingly aware of the valuable work performed by charities such as Macmillan Cancer Support and also hospices. Her involvement with her local day-care hospice when living in Derbyshire inspired her to explore ways in which to share the positive philosophy she discovered there. As she researched, she realised she was uniquely qualified to help those who are related or closely connected to cancer sufferers. They are also affected by the diagnosis of the disease, and yet support is so often lacking for them.

Anne gained her expertise through personal experience. Her mother was diagnosed with secondary brain tumours in early 1991. The months that followed to her death were extremely challenging – in spite of the fact that Anne had very little physical input to her care. Each of those who loved her had a different perspective, their own experience. And all found the process very traumatic. Whilst practical support was available, emotionally the family just 'got through' the experience as best they could.

Anne then undertook many years of personal development, during which she gradually made sense of her experiences. When her mother-in-law was diagnosed with breast cancer, Anne was older, wiser and able to truly support her in whatever ways she needed. This time the outcome was happier, and Anne had coped much better with the stress in her own life. In sharing the insights she has gained over these years, she is finding her own sense of purpose in encouraging others to find their own lessons in the challenge that has been put before them.

Lightning Source UK Ltd.
Milton Keynes UK
UKOW050758170812

197685UK00001B/64/P